# YOUR
# BRAIN ON
# NATURE

# YOUR
# BRAIN ON
# NATURE

## THE SCIENCE OF NATURE'S
## INFLUENCE ON YOUR HEALTH,
## HAPPINESS, AND VITALITY

EVA M. SELHUB, MD
ALAN C. LOGAN, ND

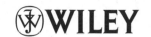

John Wiley & Sons Canada, Ltd.

**Library and Archives Canada Cataloguing in Publication**

Selhub, Eva M.
   Your brain on nature : the science of nature's influence on your health, happiness, and vitality / Eva M. Selhub and Alan C. Logan.

Includes index.
Also issued in electronic format.
ISBN 978-1-118-10674-7

   1. Brain.   2. Human beings—Effect of environment on.   3. Technology—Health aspects.
I.   Logan, Alan C., 1967–  II.   Title.

QP376.S44 2012          612.8'2          C2012-900904-0

ISBN 978-1-118-10674-7 (pbk); ISBN 978-1-118-11449-0 (ebk); ISBN 978-1-118-11450-6 (ebk); ISBN 978-1-118-11451-3 (ebk)

**Production Credits**
Managing Editor: Alison Maclean
Executive Editor: Robert Hickey
Production Editor: Pauline Ricablanca
Cover Design & Cover Art: Adrian So
Composition: Thomson Digital
Printer: Friesens Corporation

John Wiley & Sons Canada, Ltd.
6045 Freemont Blvd.
Mississauga, Ontario
L5R 4J3

Printed in Canada

1 2 3 4 5 FC 16 15 14 13 12

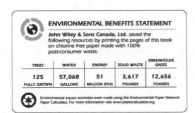

ENVIRONMENTAL BENEFITS STATEMENT

John Wiley & Sons Canada, Ltd. saved the following resources by printing the pages of this book on chlorine free paper made with 100% post-consumer waste.

| TREES | WATER | ENERGY | SOLID WASTE | GREENHOUSE GASES |
|---|---|---|---|---|
| 125 | 57,068 | 51 | 3,617 | 12,656 |
| FULLY GROWN | GALLONS | MILLION BTUs | POUNDS | POUNDS |

Environmental impact estimates were made using the Environmental Paper Network Paper Calculator. For more information visit www.papercalculator.org.

*This book is dedicated to Woodsy Owl and all individuals who have worked tirelessly to preserve nature, to balance protection with access and opportunity for nature engagement, and to raise awareness of nature's importance to human health.*

# Contents

# Introduction

Humanity's relationship with nature, a never-dull affair based on both fear and attraction, spans more than 2 million years. Our ancestors grew to understand the natural landscape, figuring out over time how to maximize their ability to secure the factors that sustained life and minimize the multiple threats to it. They grew to respect nature, balancing the understanding that nature can bite, sting, poison, maim, and kill, with an awe and appreciation of what the natural world could offer to promote health of mind and body.

Throughout the ages, and across cultures, philosophers, poets, nature writers, and outdoor enthusiasts have extolled the mentally rejuvenating and uplifting power of nature. But what of the science? To what extent is the 2-million-year relationship with the natural environment imprinted in our neurons, and to what extent does nature immersion and deprivation work for and against the individual?

In our contemporary age of science and technology, researchers have finally turned their attention toward the evaluation of these enthusiastic claims related to the medical aspects of nature. What started as a trickle of scientific inquiry in the 1970s has transformed into a formidable body of research, with many of the most startling research findings published within just the last 36 months. Scientific researchers are investigating nature's role in mental health at a time when humans are more distanced from the natural world than ever before, an environmental context in which humans are increasingly becoming part of the machine. Humans have long demonstrated a pronounced ability to use technology to conquer, control, and adapt to our natural environments. Our earliest ancestors used fire and crafted cutting and hunting tools, clothing, and shelters. Since then, technology and man's mastery over the natural environment have developed at an astonishing rate. As far back as a century ago, writers were concerned that industrialization had placed a machine in the garden, one capable of dramatically changing our natural world. Today, not only has the machine taken over the garden but there are also legitimate fears that there is now only a bit of the garden left within the machine.

This should be of great concern: natural environments offer unbelievable benefits for our health. As neuroscience develops at a rapid pace, researchers are uncovering functional aspects of the intricate anatomy and physiology of the human brain, allowing them to have a clearer picture of the true depths to which environmental factors influence cognitive and mental health. So far, the results suggest that we have completely underestimated the way in which the human brain is influenced by its physical environment and, in particular, by the elements of the natural worlds of water, vegetation, and animals. (And for our purposes, this is what we mean when we refer to nature: the nonbuilt, nonsynthetic environment—sights, sounds, aromas, rivers, oceans, plants, animals, and light in as close a form as possible to that from which we evolved.)

Undoubtedly, technology has allowed for the strength and global spread of our species, and as such, it has largely escaped meaningful criticism and broad public discourse. But today's easy access and prolonged exposure to gadgetry is leading to nature deprivation, and what is lost through that might be far more detrimental than what is gained. We want to differentiate personal gadgetry—TVs, smartphones, tablets, and home PCs—from a long list of more meaningful technology, from life-saving medical technology to freshness-preserving refrigerators. While not anti-technology (or Luddites), and with the understanding that technology has increased safety and convenience in immeasurable ways, we are unabashed screen-time critics. Nature withdrawal is being driven, at least in part, by the lure of info-entertainment-rich commercial screens—the attraction of the screen and indoor video games, so-called videophilia, is very strong.

Less contact with nature, particularly in one's young years, appears to remove a layer of protection against psychological stress and opportunity for cognitive rejuvenation. Japanese research suggests also that nature deprivation may have wide-ranging effects on the immune system. In the big picture, our turn away from nature is associated with less empathy and attraction to nature and, in turn, less interest in environmental efforts related to nature. An obvious concern is that a massive withdrawal from nature will immunize us against empathic views of nature. Sustainability of the planet is not merely about being a good citizen and recycling; it is ultimately about maintaining an intimate relationship with nature. Research shows that in order to truly care about "being green," one must actually have meaningful exposure to nature.

*Your Brain on Nature* offers readers a chance to more fully understand the impact that nature (or a lack of nature) has on individuals and society and suggests ways in which they can bring nature back into their lives. We present research showing that exposure to nature-based environments is associated with lower blood pressure and reduced levels of the stress hormone cortisol (and other objective markers of stress). And that exposure to nature is also responsible for higher levels of activity in the branch of the nervous system responsible for calming us down (the parasympathetic branch).

We introduce you to a variety of ways to help you reconnect with nature:

- Practicing *shinrin-yoku* (a Japanese concept that literally translates as "forest air bathing," or walking while taking in the forest environment with all senses). Multiple scientific studies have been published on shinrin-yoku in the last several years. These studies make it clear that even urban forests can have the effect of a mental tonic.

- Keeping plants in your office, which might help with your attentiveness.
- Employing essential oils derived from nature, which can help you stay alert, or settle down for a rejuvenating rest.
- Exercising outdoors, which has been proven to be more beneficial for the body and mind.
- Owning a pet (most notably a dog or cat). The connections between pet ownership and physical and mental health are evident: pets can lower our stress hormones and improve other measurements of stress physiology.
- Grounding the mind with gardening and away-from-it-all excursions. Horticulture and wilderness therapies can be effective interventions for mental health issues.
- Following a Mediterranean diet and whole-food nutrition, which will return you to the foods on which humans evolved to thrive.

Finally, we round out the discussion by taking a look at the historical roots and current opportunities for change provided by ecopsychology and ecopsychiatry. Allied health professionals working under the umbrella term of "ecotherapy" are educating other healthcare providers, the public, and influential leaders on the importance of mindful nature interaction for personal and planetary health. Ecotherapists, we believe, will be a driving force for broad change.

This is far from a pop-psychology book, and at times there is considerable depth to the discussions. (We examined thousands of sources, both historical and contemporary, and our detailed list of references is available online for your review at www.yourbrainonnature.com.) Although we try to keep the material as straightforward and readable as possible, there needs to be some depth to the discussions so that we can demonstrate why powering down and going outside has long-term implications for humans and the survival of the planet itself. Our in-depth analysis with historical perspective provides a true understanding of the mechanism through which nature contact can influence personal, community, and global health.

The combined authorship of a conventionally trained physician and a naturopath is uncommon; we hope that our differing trainings and backgrounds provide a unique and comprehensive perspective. Physician attention to this topic is rare, but the application of the healing power of nature (*vis medicatrix naturae* in Latin) should be embraced by all players in the health-care arena, conventional, complementary, or otherwise. As cities worldwide expand, the importance of green space in human health is an issue of common ground for all. We hope that this book serves as a template for shared discussion and decision making at a time when we are being overwhelmed with gadgetry. We can envision an optimistic future accompanying the inevitable bulging of global urban centers, and that bright future involves more green in more places.

Yours in health!

Eva M. Selhub, MD          Alan C. Logan, ND

# 1

## Nature on the Brain: From Ancient Intuition to Magnetic Resonance Imaging

*Man is an outdoor animal. He toils at desks and talks of ledgers and parlors and art galleries but the endurance that brought him these was developed by rude ancestors, whose claim to kinship he would scorn and whose vitality he has inherited and squandered. He is what he is by reason of countless ages of direct contact with nature.*

—James H. McBride, MD, *Journal of the American Medical Association,* 1902

$A$s children, both of us grew up in households where time spent in nature was encouraged, and our current memories tell us that such times in the great outdoors were filled with curiosity, fascination, and discovery, as well as with calm, joy, and happiness. The fragrance of pine and flowers; the sounds of rushing creeks, waterfalls, and ocean waves breaking; and the sights of fireflies and other interesting animals captured our minds. As time passed, our responsibilities and adulthood pursuits left less time for nature immersion. The recognition and instant recall of nature's benefits would be obscured by our own efforts to advance in a technologically driven world. Our individual stressors, personal anxieties, and the overwhelming demands of contemporary life would ultimately bring us back to the medicinal aspects of nature, to our current investigation of the scientific validity of those child-hood memories.

The pattern of our close relationship to nature in childhood development and subsequent distancing through early adulthood in many ways mirrors the development of Western civilization: as our society has progressed, we have moved away from nature, placing greater importance on technological pursuits and our own creations. Mounting scientific evidence is revealing, however, that by pushing ourselves away from nature, we humans not only have distanced ourselves from crisis-level environmental concerns but are risking losing contact with one of the most vital mental health tools imaginable—nature. Both of us are fortunate to have nature-filled childhood memories to draw on. The experiences allow us to recognize and appreciate the value of nature and the importance of environmental protection. Yet, what might happen if those memories didn't exist? What would happen if our childhood experiences and relationship to the natural world were to be shaped exclusively by pixilated images and time spent in front of a screen? By denying ourselves nature, we humans risk denying a vital part of our heritage, a truth that, ironically, through advances in medical technology, we are now able to see more clearly.

## Biophilia—Humanity's Vital Bond with Nature

Humanity's historical contact with nature has left an indelible mark, a driving force for us to have an affinity for all things living (plants and animals alike). Our connection to nature is right there in our DNA: that's the essence of the biophilia hypothesis. "Biophilia" was originally defined in early 1900s' medical dictionaries as the instinct for self-preservation or the instinctual drive to stay alive. In the 1980s, Harvard biologist Edward O. Wilson proposed that biophilia is an "innately emotional affiliation of human beings to other living organisms." Wilson didn't see humanity's affiliation with nature as stemming from individual experience or romantic notions, nor as a by-product of North America's wilderness attraction. Rather, he saw biophilia as a common thread spanning across cultures, a phenomenon that has been confirmed to some degree by various groups of scientists who have determined that the preference for certain aspects of nature is culturally universal—landscapes that provide trees (but not too densely packed), views that afford a vista or some degree of predator surveillance, the presence of fresh water, and a rich variety of plants and animals.

Wilson's definition of "biophilia" extended to the emotional plane. He observed that nature uniquely influenced the human mind, having the potential to influence the matters that mental-health-care providers concern themselves with: cognitions and behaviors. Wilson's expanded view still fulfills the original definition of "biophilia" because these innate cognitive and behavioral reactions to the natural world ensure self-preservation: they draw us close to adequate water, nutrition, and shelter, and ensure that we flee from a predatory beast. Evidence suggests, for example, that we are born with a predisposition to fear poisonous reptiles and spiders—having never seen these creatures. Experimental studies have shown that a physiological stress response is set in motion even when an individual is consciously unaware of the threat. The researchers use clever masking techniques whereby they show pictures of the potentially threatening stimuli (such as a spider) to a test subject so rapidly (for only 30 milliseconds) in sequence with neutral images that the individual does not consciously perceive the threatening stimulus when queried. A pronounced stress response to these threatening stimuli can be observed, and conditioning studies show that these "ancient" fears become easily ingrained and more resistant to elimination, as opposed to modern threats such as guns, or neutral objects such as mushrooms or flowers.

Researchers at the University of California, Santa Barbara identified further support for the biophilia hypothesis when they challenged test subjects to detect changes in photographic scenes of animals compared with images of vehicles and inanimate objects. Given that people face cars every day, and they pose a far greater threat in contemporary life than animals do, one might expect the subjects to be better attuned to the images of the vehicles. Yet, it seems that the priority in visually monitoring animals, a critical skill for the hunter-gatherer, is still alive and well in the modern screen-toting adult—a reality that does not serve well while trying to walk and text in a metro area. This was something that Wilson had proposed regarding biophilia: contact with nature shaped the human brain and, as such, it was pre-equipped for a specific view, one that would "persist from generation to generation, atrophied and fitfully manifested in the artificial new environments into which technology has catapulted humanity." There may be some atrophy in our modern world, but the biophilic response remains—in underappreciated ways.

Recent studies conducted in 2010 by University of Virginia psychologists have underscored just how innate humanity's responses to nature are: infants demonstrate signs of fear when exposed to natural threats they've never been culturally groomed to fear. Of note is that the subliminal exposure to spiders fires up activity in the amygdalae (singular amygdala; these are two almond-sized and -shaped brain structures referred to as the fear centers of the brain). While it might be amplified by social learning (and perhaps watching movies such as *Arachnophobia* at a young age), the brain-based detection of ancient nature-based threats seems to be in our genetic code. Although humanity's affiliation with nature might be amplified by social learning and romanticism, nature appears to fire up the brain just as it did in our primitive ancestors. For example, test subjects shown even a one-tenth-of-a-second glimpse of scenes of nature prefer them over urban and built scenes; indeed, a reflection of the innate preference comes from the finding that the more rapid the presentation of the nature images within other environmental scenes, the more the nature scenes are preferred over the built.

## Nature: An Ancient Cure Abandoned

Healers within various medical systems, from ayurveda of the Indian subcontinent to traditional Chinese medicine, have long advocated nature exposure as a form of medicine. Within these healing systems, elements of nature—mountains, trees, plants, and bodies of water within natural settings—are considered to be filled with an energy, a vital force that could be transferred to people in the promotion of health. As humans began to make a transition from rural life to urban civilizations, an even greater emphasis was placed on taking advantage of the medicinal effects of nature. For example, records of early Roman philosophers and physicians, such as Cornelius Celsus, show that walking in gardens, exposure to rooms filled with light, staying close to water, and other nature-based activities were effective components of standardized plans to improve mental health and sleep.

The notion of unspoilt nature as a mental healer gained popularity in North America in the mid- to late 19th century. Once again it was spurred on by the rapid expansion of cities and growing concerns that the industrial revolution, with its dimly lit, poorly ventilated work-places and crowded residences, was contributing to mental distress. In the 1800s, writers such as Henry David Thoreau and naturalist John Muir voiced their concerns about urban life and described nature as essential to well-being. Thoreau described nature as a calming tonic and creativity booster, a place where "my nerves are steadied, my senses and my mind do their office." Muir reported that "tired, nerve-shaken, over-civilized people" could experience an awakening while wandering in wilderness. In his 1898 address at the annual meeting of the American Medical Association, physician Frederic S. Thomas linked higher rates of mental health problems with the stresses of modern civilization. Overstimulation, noise, smoke, and stench were, he felt, acting upon inherited susceptibilities.

Frederick Law Olmsted, a landscape architect and key player in the development of parks throughout the United States, was motivated by his view that parks had a beneficial impact on positive mental health. His 1865 federal report on the status of Yosemite National Park stated, "If we analyze the operation of scenes of beauty upon the mind, and consider the intimate relation of the mind upon the nervous system and the whole physical economy, the action and reaction which constantly occurs between bodily and mental conditions, the reinvigoration which results from such scenes is readily comprehended." The report noted that immersion in nature is favorable to health, vigor, and intellect and "that it not only gives pleasure for the time being but increases the subsequent capacity for happiness and the means of securing happiness." While obviously not proposed as a cure for mental illness, nature-based recreation was described in the report as a means of reducing "mental and nervous excitability, moroseness, melancholy, or irascibility" that would diminish optimal mental functioning.

As North American cities expanded rapidly, medical doctors began to prescribe nature exposure as a means of reducing stress and improving mental outlook. This practice was not based on scientific evidence; it was a return to the intuitive recommendations of the ancient healers. However, contemporary research was connecting anxiety and depression to the stress of modern urban life, so it seemed plausible that a break from these pressures would be a safe prescription. A thriving industry of privately funded sanitariums and health resorts, all set deep within natural settings, took flight. The very names of these sanitariums implied a retreat to nature: The Pines, The Highlands, Lake View, River View, Crest View, Grand View, Walnut Lodge, Blue Hills, River Crest, and Glen Springs, to name just a few of the hundreds advertised within countless turn-of-the-19th-century medical journals. The owners of these establishments, and the physicians who worked within them, provided services for the treatment of mild nervous diseases and the stress-related fatigue diagnosis *du jour*, neurasthenia. Practically every ad boasted of beautiful scenery, pine forests, and charming walks. One advertisement, for The Pines, even talked of how the grounds were "rolling and diversified in character." These retreats recruited their attendees from the well-heeled urbanites and lured them to greenery. Those who weren't quite flush with cash could find an oasis in newly created metro parks, including New York's Central Park, designed by Olmsted, an individual who advocated that such urban escapes would promote mental relaxation for users.

Within the medical profession during the early 1900s there was largely an acceptance of—and in some quarters enthusiasm about—the beneficial effects of the nature retreats. The anecdotal notion was that nature could have a medicinal effect, providing a tonic for the brain as it dealt with a world that was becoming increasingly complex. Along with writing out prescriptions for some time in nature, physicians were making note that a sedentary and indoor lifestyle was at odds with our human lineage. From urban-park planners to medical doctors, all hypothesized that nature is in us, it has shaped us, and even though we may turn away, we do so at our own peril. The industrial revolution was changing the world in rapid fashion, and physicians such as James McBride, whose quotation opened this chapter, were trying to raise awareness about the growing disconnect with nature.

A variety of cultural, economic, and scientific changes put an end to the sanitarium boom. Even though there was some level of acceptance among the medical profession, and few would challenge the notion that man is indeed, as James McBride informed his colleagues, "an outdoor animal," the message was losing its way. The scientific basis for the existence of these mental retreats was extremely limited. As the cultural pendulum swung toward evidentiary validation, the assumed benefits of such institutions—exercise, whole-food diets, sunshine, open air, hydrotherapy, immersion in nature—as a means of helping nervous afflictions were all lumped in with pseudoscientific patent medicines and baldness cures. In short, doctors and scientists began to distance themselves from such soft notions that nature contact was in itself a vital force. As the automobile and suburban sprawl took over, the half-page advertisements for the Glen Springs Sanitarium gave way to full-page advertisements for the antianxiety drug meprobamate (or Miltown, the first synthesized, brand-name version of it) and other chemical means of dealing with modern stressors. Some of these now-abandoned sanitariums, the buildings being reclaimed by trees and shrubs, remain as haunting memories of yesteryear, of a time when purposeful time in nature was *the* prescription.

## Nature and Stress Physiology

The notion that nature scenes can influence psychological well-being and stress physiology remained largely untested until Roger S. Ulrich decided to pay it some attention in 1979. A few years earlier, Ulrich, as a geography PhD student, had found that residents around Ann Arbor, Michigan, were typically skipping an expressway and taking a longer and slower route to the major mall simply because it was reported to be more scenic. They were sacrificing time and gas money to take a longer route, and he wanted to know what might be motivating that seemingly consistent decision. Ulrich wanted to dig deeper and have a look at the psychological variables that might explain how the aesthetics of natural landscapes can influence human behavior.

He decided to examine the mental influences of nature scenes on stressed students. After taking a required one-hour course exam in a windowless room, 46 students volunteered to do some psychological tests and then view about 50 slides. After answering the questions, the students were split into two groups: one viewed slides of natural settings devoid of buildings, and the other group looked at urban buildings (retail and industrial) that did not have graffiti or litter present. Images of people and animals were excluded from the slides. The psychological testing showed that although the students were indeed a bit stressed and frazzled after their one-hour exam, their divergent mental states and outlook after viewing the two types of environmental scenes were striking. The nature scenes increased positive affect—feelings of affection, playfulness, friendliness, and elation were elevated in the group that viewed various nature scenes. Not so for those who viewed the urban scenes. Those views significantly cultivated one emotion in these stressed students: sadness. The nature scenes tended to decrease feelings of anger and aggression, and urban scenes tended to increase them. Given the ability of stress to drag down health, and positive mental outlook to buffer stress and promote health, the implication of this report was clearly enormous. Still, it required validation; in particular, scientifically valid markers of the body's stress response would help bolster the case for nature.

Encouraged, Ulrich moved forward from the initial subjective testing to examine how nature scenes might influence stress physiology and even brain activity. He set up a similar experiment with unstressed healthy adults, although this time he also used an electroencephalograph (EEG) apparatus to measure brain activity. Sure enough, the team discovered that viewing scenes of nature was associated with higher alpha wave amplitudes, which is a good thing. Higher alpha wave activity is associated with increased serotonin production. Serotonin is a chemical that operates within the nervous system. Almost all antidepressant medications are thought to work by enhancing the availability of serotonin for use in nerve cell communication, hence its moniker of "the happy chemical." When we turn the dial down on hyperarousal and calm sets in, as is the case in meditative states, higher alpha wave activity is noted. On the other hand, anxiety is associated with lower alpha wave amplitude and enhanced activity of beta waves.

Ulrich followed this up with another study to assess the ability of nature scenes to influence stress physiology via heart, skin, and muscle readings—including pulse transit time and electrocardiogram (EKG), skin conductance (sweat on the skin, which is influenced by the stress response), and muscle tension via electromyography (EMG). Some 120 undergraduate students watched a stressful video related to workplace errors with tragic consequences (entitled *It Didn't Have to Happen*). Immediately after the 10-minute video, the subjects watched another 10-minute video containing either urban scenery (retail, commercial, with and without traffic and crowds) or natural scenery (trees, vegetation, with and without water). The objective measurements showed that those who watched nature scenes had a more rapid and complete recovery from the stress caused by watching *It Didn't Have to Happen*. Nature acted as a sort of visual valium; the nature scenes fostered positive thoughts and lowered anger and aggression post-stressor. For many of the participants, not only did the nature scenes offset the effects of the stressful video but their reports of positive mental outlook were higher than their pretest scores.

Additional work from Ulrich and his team has shown that nature scenes reduced physiological markers of stress among 872 blood donors. In this study, all donors sat in the same waiting room over the course of a three-month period. The only variable manipulated was the programming shown on the wall-mounted TV: some days the TV was off, some days it was playing standard daytime television, some days it was rolling scenes of an urban environment, and on the other days it was displaying nature scenes. Blood pressure and pulse rates showed that stress was lowest with the TV off. In other words, the common assumption that more TVs and daytime TV programming—news, soaps, talk shows—are helping patients in the waiting room is nothing more than another screen legend. However, if the TV must be on, nature scenes displayed on the screen were associated with lower stress compared with urban and daytime programming.

Ulrich's pioneering work using objective testing has been supported by recent investigations by international researchers:

- Older adults in a residential care center in Texas were shown to produce lower levels of the stress hormone cortisol after engagement in the same mental activities (such as scanning photo books and making observations about the environment) within a garden setting as opposed to an indoor classroom.
- The presence of plants in a room, particularly flowering plants, can enhance recovery from the stress induced by an emotional video and quickly bring EEG beta wave activity back to normal, researchers at Kansas State University found.

- A group from Taiwan reported that a variety of nature scenes—streams, valleys, river terraces, orchards, forests, farms, and bodies of water—have therapeutic effects based on the same objective markers of EEG, EMG, and skin conductance. For example, rural farm scenes are associated with higher alpha wave activity, particularly in the right part of the brain, which has been linked with creativity. Forest scenes and nature scenes with water promote alpha wave activity and decrease heart rate. On the contrary, an increase in muscular tension has been associated with an urban view.
- Japanese researchers evaluated physiological stress markers in 119 adults who transplanted nonflowering plants from one pot to another. Compared with adults who simply filled pots with soil, the individuals working with the plants had higher alpha wave production immediately after the task; they also had less muscular tension as measured by EMG, as well as subjective reductions in fatigue.
- Researchers in Japan have also replicated via EKG the finding of lowered heart rate while viewing nature scenes for 20 minutes versus viewing urban scenes. A 2004 study of patients with mental illness showed that the presence of green plants (ficus species) lowers blood pressure and heart rate, and the plants also amplified alpha wave activity.

These studies all represent major steps forward in the scientific evaluation of the brain on nature. Still, it is not nearly enough to make a convincing argument that nature is influencing us in more ways than we might even fathom. On the one hand, it might seem impressive that merely viewing nature scenes could have such profound effects on stress physiology and mood, yet it remains an open question as to what the effects might be if we are truly immersed in nature, walking through it and breathing it in. It is only when we add in the abundance of research from the members of the Japanese Society of Forest Medicine that a picture truly begins to emerge.

# Shinrin-Yoku—Forest Bathing

*It is not so much for its beauty that the forest makes a*
*claim upon men's hearts, as for that subtle something,*
*that quality of air that emanation from old trees, that*
*so wonderfully changes and renews a weary spirit.*

—Robert Louis Stevenson

Among the many reasons to preserve what is left of our ancient forests, the mental aspects stand tall. The notion that forests have a special place in the realm of public health, including an ability to refresh the weary, is not a new one. Medical doctors, including Franklin B. Hough, reported in early U.S. medical journals that forests have a "cheerful and tranquilizing influence which they exert upon the mind, more especially when worn down by mental labor." Individuals report that forests are the perfect landscape to cultivate what are called transcendent experiences—these are unforgettable moments of extreme happiness, of attunement to that outside the self, and moments that are ultimately perceived as very important to the individual.

In 1982, the Forest Agency of the Japanese government premiered its shinrin-yoku plan. In Japanese *shinrin* means forest, and *yoku,* although it has several meanings, refers here to a "bathing, showering or basking in." More broadly, it is defined as "taking in, in all of our senses, the forest atmosphere." The program was established to encourage the populace to get out into nature, to literally bathe the mind and body in greenspace, and take advantage of public-owned forest networks as a means of promoting health. Some 64 percent of Japan is occupied by forest, so there is ample opportunity to escape the megacities that dot its landscape.

Undoubtedly, the Japanese have had a centuries-old appreciation of the therapeutic value of nature—including its old-growth forests; however, the term *shinrin-yoku* is far from ancient. It began really as a marketing term, coined by Tomohide Akiyama in 1982 during his brief stint as director of Japan's Forest Agency. The initial shinrin-yoku plan of 30 years ago was based solely on the ingrained perception that spending time in nature, particularly on lush Japanese forest trails, would do the mind and body good. That changed in 1990 when Dr. Yoshifumi Miyazaki of Chiba University was trailed by a film crew from the Japanese Broadcasting Corporation (NHK) as he conducted a small study in the beautiful forests of Yakushima. It was a test of shinrin-yoku, and NHK wanted to be there. Yakushima was chosen because it is home to Japan's most heralded forests. The area contains some of Japan's most pristine forests, including those of select cedar trees that are over 1,000 years old. Miyazaki reported that a level of physical activity (40 minutes of walking) in the cedar forest equivalent to that done indoors in a laboratory was associated with improved mood and feelings of vigor. This in itself is hardly a revelation, but he backed up the subjective reports by the findings of lower levels of the stress hormone cortisol in subjects after forest walks compared with those who took laboratory walks. It was the first hint that a walk in a forest might not be the same as a walk in a different environmental setting.

Since then, university and government researchers have collaborated on detailed investigations, including projects to evaluate physiological markers while subjects spend time in the forest. The research team from Chiba University, Center for Environment, Health and Field Services has collected psychological and physiological data on some 500 adults who have engaged in shinrin-yoku, and a separate group from Kyoto has published research involving another 500 adults. These studies have confirmed that spending time within a forest setting can reduce psychological stress, depressive symptoms, and hostility, while at the same time improving sleep and increasing both vigor and a feeling of liveliness. These subjective changes match up nicely with objective results reported in nearly a dozen studies involving 24 forests—lower levels of cortisol and lower blood pressure and pulse rate. In addition, studies showed increased heart rate variability, which is a good thing because it means the circulatory system can respond well to stress and can detect a dominance of the "calming" branch of the nervous system (the parasympathetic nervous system).

---

### Just the Right Amount of Trees

Research has shown that the emotions of pleasure and happiness are elevated with an increase in tree density within specific settings, even in urban settings. The bigger and denser the trees, the higher the scenic beauty scores—up to a point. If trees are too tightly packed—if a trail is too narrow or obscured—the scene becomes foreboding and fear will be increased.

Similarly, lining one's walls with wood might be too much of a good thing. Japanese researchers have found the sweet spot for just the right amount of wood on the floor and walls in an interior environment—somewhere between 30 and 40 percent of surface area. This percentage has the highest rating of relaxation and is linked to lower physiological stress markers (blood pressure and pulse rate). If you go all out and wood panel the entire room, like many a North American split-level ranch basement circa 1970, the stress markers can increase!

---

Adding to the strength of the research, in many of the studies, the objective measurements were also recorded in urban environments as a means of comparison. Here, the researchers controlled for physical activity, time of day, temperature, average hours of sunlight, and other factors. In other words, they weren't stacking the deck by recording the objective measurements in rainy and cold urban settings compared with sunny and warm forest environments. In one study, the researchers went so far as to bring an instrument capable of measuring brain activity out into the urban and forest settings. The time-resolved spectroscopy system (TRSS) device allows for a reading of oxygen use in the brain via the reflection of near–infrared light off red blood cells. The Japanese researchers found that 20 minutes of shinrin-yoku (compared with 20 minutes in an urban setting) altered cerebral blood flow in a manner that indicated a state of relaxation. More specifically, the total hemoglobin (as found in red blood cells) was decreased in the area of the prefrontal cortex while in the forest setting. Hemoglobin levels are jacked up in this area during antici-pation of a threat (stress) and after periods of intense mental and physical work—complex equations, computer testing, video game playing, exercise to exhaustion. So essentially, a decrease in levels means the brain is taking a time-out while in the forest. Although sedatives are also known to reduce activity in this area of the brain, they can have detrimental influences in cognition. (We discuss in the next chapter how the restorative influences of nature actually increase cognitive abilities.)

Stress hormones can compromise immune defense; in particular, the activities of frontline defenders, such as antiviral natural killer cells, are suppressed by stress hormones. Since forest bathing can lower stress hormone production and elevate mood states, it's not surprising that it also influences markers of immune system strength. Qing Li and colleagues from the Nippon Medical School showed that forest bathing (either a day trip or a couple of hours daily over three days) can have a long-lasting influence on immune markers relative to city trips. Specifically, there were marked increases in the number of natural killer cells, increases in the functional activity of these antiviral cells, and increases in the amount of intracellular anticancer proteins. The changes were noted at a significant level for a full week after the trip. The improvements in immune functioning were associated with lower urinary stress hormones while in nature. None of this was observed during or after the comparison city trips. As mentioned, the reduction in stress is almost certainly at play in the improvement of immune defenses. However, the natural chemicals secreted by evergreen trees, collectively known as phytoncide, have also been associated with improvements in the activity of our front-line immune defenders. Li has measured the amount of phytoncide in the air during the studies and correlated the content to improvements in immune functioning. This is an interesting finding in the context of the century-old reports on the success of the so-called forest cure in tuberculosis treatment. In the mid- to late 1800s, physicians Peter Detweiler and Hermann Brehmer set up sanatoriums in Germany's pine forests, as did Edward Trudeau in the Adirondack forests of New York. All reported the benefit of the forest air; indeed, contrary to expectations, the results seemed to be magnified when the forest air trapped moisture. There was speculation among the physicians of the time that pine trees secreted a healing balm into the air, and in yet another twist of the shinrin-yoku studies, the existence of an unseen airborne healer is being revealed. We discuss this in more detail later.

Shinrin-yoku is alive and well today; the word has entered the Japanese lexicon. At present there are 44 locations approved as "forest therapy bases." These sites have been not only the subject of human research indicating benefits to stress physiology; a team of experts from the Japanese Forest Therapy Executive Committee ensures other criteria are met before designation, including accessibility, accommodation (if remote), cultural landmarks, historical sites, variety of food choices, and comfort stations. Chiba University's Miyazaki, who played a massive role in taking shinrin-yoku from a throwback marketing concept to credible preventive medicine intervention, continues to perform research and is now looking at the physiological effects of time spent in Tokyo's major urban parks.

## Plants, Pain, and Sickness

In the midst of performing his physiology studies, Ulrich published a landmark study in the prestigious journal *Science* in 1984. He collected records from a single suburban Pennsylvania hospital from 1972 to 1981. He was very specific in what he examined—adults who had undergone identical surgery to remove the gallbladder (cholecystectomy) during this time frame—and the only major distinction among the patients was the room into which they were wheeled for recovery. Rooms on one side of the hospital had windows with a view to a mini-forest, while rooms on the other side offered a dramatically different vista in the form of bricks *du rouge*. The results were quite dramatic: those who had an outdoor view to trees had significantly shorter hospital stays and fewer postsurgical complaints. They also used less-potent analgesic medications (aspirin instead of narcotics). And to top it off, their nurses made fewer negative comments in their charts—and isn't it the dream of every patient to get out of a medical setting without the words "difficult patient" inscribed into a permanent medical record?

Ulrich, now retired from Texas A&M University and living in Sweden, has recently disclosed that his own experiences helped motivate him to examine the view from the hospital windows. Bedridden for extended periods as a teen with kidney disease, Ulrich recalls that his own view to evergreen was a factor that helped his emotional state. His original scientific observations have been replicated. For example, a recent study of cardio-pulmonary patients (published in *Clinical Rehabilitation* in 2011) showed that patients who had an unobstructed view of nature self-reported higher levels of health.

Since Ulrich's original observation, there have been additional studies confirming that the mere presence of flowering and foliage plants inside a hospital room can make a difference. Specifically, in those recovering an appendectomy and randomly assigned to a room with a dozen small potted plants, the use of pain medications was significantly lower than that of their counterparts in rooms with no potted plants; they also had lower blood pressure and heart rate, and rated their pain to be much lower. As well, those who had plants in their rooms had comparatively higher energy levels, more positive thoughts, and lower levels of anxiety.

Since a view of nature or a few potted plants can influence subjective and objective measures of stress, and maybe get us out of the hospital faster, it seems likely that nature can keep us out of the infirmary to begin with. The first indication that this might be the case was in the reporting of architect Ernest Moore in 1981. In examining the annual sick records of the State Prison of Southern Michigan, he noticed there was a glaring difference in health-care utilization based on cell location. Specifically, those inmates housed in the cells facing outside to a view of green farmlands and forests had far fewer visits to the medical division than did those inmates housed in the inner half, with a view of an internal concrete yard. In addition,

- Norwegian research shows that having a plant at or within view of an office workstation significantly decreases the risk of sick leave. A 2010 study from the University of Technology, Sydney, Australia, reported that levels of anger, anxiety, depressive thoughts, and fatigue all reduced over a three-month period, and not just by a little bit—these parameters were reduced by about 40 percent, while reported stress was down by 50 percent. On the other hand, those without the stress buffer of a visible plant indicated that stress levels rose over 20 percent during the study.
- Installing plants within a radiology department of a hospital reduced short-term sick leave by 60 percent.
- Research published in 2008 in the *Journal of the Japanese Society for Horticultural Science* showed that greening select high school classrooms with potted plants for a four-month trial period significantly reduced visits to the infirmary compared with age-matched students attending classes without the visible plants.

## Neighborhood Greenness—Stress Buffer, Life Saver

Projections indicate that in less than 20 years, 75 percent of the world's population will be living in urban settings. The potential ability of a single factor to buffer against the associated daily hassles and the stress hormone cascade will have enormous implications for us and our future generations. As exciting, cutting-edge studies confirm that viewing nature scenes can put a dampener on the raging fires of stress physiology, research has also shown that access to greenspace provides a much-needed buffer against stress. Specifically, those living within a three-kilometer (almost two-mile) radius of a high amount of greenspace (as measured by the National Land Cover Classification Database) were less likely to experience the negative health impacts of stress. Among those who had experienced recent life stressors (major losses, financial problems, relationship problems, legal issues, and so on), having a more dense greenspace within a three-kilometer radius was associated with fewer health complaints compared with those with a low amount of greenspace.

A 2003 investigation involving 337 children showed higher levels of nearby nature diminished the psychological impact of stressful life events. In this case, the children, average age 9, were from five small towns in New York State. No child is immune from stress and adversity, yet when childhood hardships start to add up, they set the stage for a life filled with anxiety and depressive thoughts. Remember the fear centers of the brain, the amygdalae, the areas cooled off by nature and fired up by built urban scenes? Consider that in children who have grown up with an accumulation of stressors—major losses, violence, abuse, bullying, institutional care—the amygdalae are significantly larger, and this is accompanied by a long-term processing bias toward negativity and danger within the brain. It is not our contention that time in nature alone can undo harm done; yet, if safe neighborhood greenspace can take even some of the load off the amygdala, providing even a bit of respite from the stress cascade—and research shows that it does—then researchers and clinicians should be placing full priority on examining greenspace as a medicinal agent.

Because greenspace provides a stress buffer, and so many aspects of human health and even longevity itself are negatively influenced by stress, it follows that greenspace is a promoter of human health, vitality, and longevity. A study involving over 11,000 adults in Denmark showed that those living more than one kilometer (about half a mile) from greenspace (including forests, parks, beaches, and lakes) were 42 percent more likely to report high stress and had the worst scores on evaluations of general health, vitality, mental health, and bodily pain. Those with only 10 percent greenspace within one kilometer (0.6 miles) had a 25 percent greater risk of depression and a 30 percent greater risk of anxiety disorders versus those at the upper end of greenspace near the home. These are remarkable findings. Moreover, when researchers in the Netherlands examined medical records of 195 family physicians, they found that the annual prevalence rate of 15 of the top 24 disease states were lowest among those with the highest greenspace within a one-kilometer (0.6-mile) radius from home.

Indeed, the following four studies show that greenness is associated with lower mortality:

- Researchers at the Nippon Medical School in Japan compared data on the percentage of forest coverage in all prefectures and cancer mortality rates provided by the Ministry of Health. Even after they controlled for smoking and socioeconomic factors, higher forest coverage within prefectures provided a significant protective effect against various cancers—lung, breast, uterine, prostate, kidney, and colon cancers.
- In a U.S. study, researchers at the University of West Florida examined five years' worth of data on stroke mortality and found that geographic greenspace (measured via satellite technology) offered significant protection, while areas low in greenspace were associated with a very high risk of stroke mortality.
- In a large study involving the residents of Shanghai, researchers reported that neighborhoods with a higher proportion of parks, gardens, and other green areas were associated with a reduced risk of mortality.
- Researchers at the University of Glasgow, Scotland, compared a land-use database for greenspace and mortality records. As with the Shanghai study, they found the same association between residence in the greenest areas and lower rates of death.

As with the large Japanese study, the Scottish researchers controlled for socioeconomic differences, as the greater access to greenspace among the affluent may be a surrogate marker for the other health advantages (health-care access, nutrition, lower cumulative stress levels, lower cortisol, and so on) enjoyed by the rich. Incredibly, greenspace was reported to be a great equalizer—it could fill in, to a significant degree, the huge gap in health inequalities between the have mores and those struggling at the lower end of the economic spectrum. Among those with low income and high levels of residential greenery, the mortality differences compared with those of the affluent were minimized. However, when low income was associated with little surrounding greenspace, the health disconnect with the rich became significantly amplified. The researchers concluded that greenspace was an independent variable capable of saving thousands of lives per year in lower-income populations.

Local greenspace may be a mere surrogate marker for other health-promoting factors. Greenspace provides an obvious opportunity for physical activity and increased social connectivity. One study showed that living areas with the highest levels of greenery increased the likelihood of its residents being physically active threefold over neighborhoods with little greenery. Yet, even when researchers remove physical activity and social support from the equation, the association between greenery and positive mental health remains. Merely being in nature for brief periods—or even simply having it in our view—can reduce the stress hormone cascade and improve immune defense.

## Nature and the MRI Scanner

Although all of the research detailed so far is encouraging, it would be even more convincing if we could verify that beneath the cranium our neurons are indeed firing differently while the brain is affected by nature. Knowing that healthy adults typically report that color slides of fields and forests promote feelings of tranquility and usually assign higher ratings of perceived danger to color slides of urban settings is a positive step. However, critics might suggest that subjects who report improved mood while viewing nature scenes or walking in a forest are merely checking the "right" boxes in order to fulfill the expectations of researchers. Is the brain, deep within its undulations, really at work in a different way while immersed—at the very least visually immersed if not with our other senses—in its naturally evolved setting? The final frontier in objective testing is to go inside the brain, to visualize it, while it is on nature.

In 1899, physician Juan Breña stated that the calming and invigorating mental health benefits of forests "cannot be explained, as to its mechanism by any dogma of common medical science" and "will remain incomprehensible so long as we be without the clairvoyance necessary to enable us to penetrate the most hidden phenomena of physical life." The nature sanitariums of Breña's time were destined to fade without the required scientific confirmation. It would be a little over a century before researchers in California would bring in that strong dose of clairvoyance in the form of functional magnetic resonance imaging (fMRI), a sophisticated brain imaging technique. Their findings showed that more desirable views (aesthetically pleasing nature views, coastal vistas) were firing up a specific portion of the brain, the anterior portions of the parahippocampal gyrus, rich in opioid receptors. These opioid receptors have connections to the brain cells within the dopamine reward system and, as such, have the potential to trigger feelings of wellness and push forward the motivation required for positive behavioral modification.

This was an incredible finding, revealing that nature is like a little drop of morphine for the brain. Although best known for pain inhibition, the opioid receptors do so much more. When these receptors are activated, the response is remarkable: people are less likely to perceive themselves to stressed, they are more likely to form emotional bonds, and they tend to dwell less on negative memories, focusing instead on the positive. People with depression have been noted to have decreased brain activity in the anterior parahippocampal gyrus.

In additional research, these investigators and others reported that indoor scenes (such as an office, kitchen, hallway), compared with outdoor nature scenes (forests, water, mountains, vegetation), consistently produce a higher level of activity in a specific area of the brain involved in scene processing. In 2011 it was discovered that this area of the brain, the parahippocampal place area, is also much more active when viewing scenes depicting crowds of any sort, movie theaters, outdoor malls, supermarkets viewed from the outside, elevators, tunnels, heavy traffic, outdoor train stations, urban trains on the move, buses, bridges, and towers. Put simply, the area of the brain processing scene information is interacting with arousal and working overtime in nonnatural settings. The greater effort required to run the brain in the modern urban world can catch up with us in the form of mental fatigue. This uptick in brain effort required to process place in the indoor and outdoor human-made environments is most pronounced in those prone to anxiety.

---

### Dr. Eva's File

Jenna, 29 years old, described feeling overwhelmed and overworked, avoiding breaks and trying to focus on the stream of information on her computer screen, and crunching numbers for the big corporation she worked for. The major problem at hand was that she was making mistakes—big mistakes that her bosses were concerned about, so much so that she was put on probation. Stress was keeping her from sleeping and causing her headaches, and she found the numbers on the screen were starting to meld into mush. She could not concentrate. On further questioning, Jenna reported she spent at least 12 to 14 hours a day at the screen, without counting her smartphone or her personal computer use. Her time spent outdoors consisted of leaving her house or office to get into her car and vice versa. It was clear that among other things, Jenna was nature-deprived.

Jenna was given a prescription of taking 10-minute mindful walks— appreciating nature—at least once a day and putting a picture of her favorite nature scene next to her computer. She was instructed to take a break from the computer every 15 minutes to look at the picture.

By doing this, Jenna found that her concentration improved, as did her headaches, and her stress level lowered. She also realized that hers was not the right job for her.

Researchers in Korea peered into the brain via fMRI in an effort to truly see how urban scenes and nature scenes can activate certain areas of the brain. In two separate studies, Korean researchers used fMRI to assess brain activation patterns while subjects viewed nature-based scenery (mountains, forests) or urban scenery. In the first study, viewing the urban scenes resulted in pronounced activity in the amygdala and anterior temporal pole. The amygdala is referred to as an ancient part of the brain; it has been with us for as long as we have evolved with nature—and it's what is fired up when infants were exposed in testing to images of spiders, as described earlier. It is active in response to danger, including environmental threats, as well as to aversive stimuli and situations requiring snap judgment. Overactivity of the amygdala has been linked to impulsivity and anxiety. Furthermore, chronic stress and the stress hormone cortisol itself may promote amygdala activity. Once it is in an overactive state, we tend to selectively prioritize the memorization of negative events and experiences. This becomes a vicious cycle: the world looks a bit more scary and depressing, and our dominant memories confirm it to be true. In other words, once the amygdala is amped-up on a regular basis, it fuels the brain's fear pathways and short-circuits the areas that would otherwise dampen amygdala activity. The good news is that, over time, we can win back control of the rogue amygdala with awareness of our thought processes and by placing ourselves in environments that turn down the dial on the amygdala. With a mindful shift in the direction of positive mental outlook, emphasizing a preponderance of positive emotions, rather than negative emotions (more joy, contentment, vitality, interest, and love; less anger, resentment, guilt, fear, shame, and melancholy), we can rein in the amygdala. And this is where nature can play a role.

In that first study, the Korean researchers noted that the urban scenes also affected the anterior temporal pole, which is associated with negative subjective emotional responses such as anger and depression. Tellingly, the nature scenes produced a pronounced activity in two brain centers: the anterior cingulate and the insula.

Increased activity in both of these areas is associated with heightened empathy. Greater activity in the anterior cingulate is associated with emotional stability and a positive mental outlook, while less than normal brain activity there has been linked to attention deficits. Activity in the insula is associated with love. Urban scenes did not influence activity in the anterior cingulate or the insula.

The second fMRI study produced largely the same results. The design was the same: participants viewed rural and urban scenes for two minutes each, followed by a 30-second rest. To minimize the influence of a wandering mind among subjects (i.e., to prevent them from thinking about what's for dinner or how high their cable TV bill might be), the photographs were presented in fairly rapid fashion: every one and a half seconds a new photo was shown. This was not an exercise in contemplative evaluation of art; this was about tapping into the ancient portions of the brain to see how they might auto-react. Once again the researchers observed marked amygdala activity when the subjects viewed the urban scenes. This time the nature scenes promoted greater activity in the basal ganglia, an area known to be activated in response to happy faces and in recollection of happy memories. Interestingly, the nature scenes also activated the areas of the brain governing addictions and rewards, suggesting that there is hope that nature can still trump the screen if only we would let it.

Other university-based brain imaging investigations are now being planned, and some will incorporate psychological testing to determine how viewing nature and urban scenes might interact with mental outlook and pro-environmental behavior. The most recent investigation using fMRI showed that rural scenery activated the brain areas associated with positive emotions and happiness, while urban scenery produced enhanced activity in three key areas implicated in anxiety and arousal. Indeed, the urban scenes caused an uptick in activity in an area known to be active in states of anger. These early indicators of our brain on nature—although inside a sophisticated brain imaging machine—are certainly in line with the emerging neuroimaging results of psychologists and neuroscientists who have been working together in the realm of positive psychology. These researchers are trying to map out a so-called happy brain—the areas of the brain that are predominant when people are happy in the moment or report happiness in their day-to-day lives.

---

### The Urban Amygdala

Decades of research show that there are mental health consequences of life in the big city—the risk of anxiety and/or depression is up to 40 percent higher compared with residence in rural settings. Using sophisticated brain imaging, Korean researchers found that healthy adults viewing urban scenes had a significant increase in activity of the amygdala. This was not evident when the participants viewed nature scenes. In 2011, a Germany study used fMRI with the added twist of intentionally stressing their subjects in the experimental setting. They showed that urbanites, or those with a long history of urban living, are much more likely to have pronounced activity of the amygdala when they are perceived to be stressed by other humans. All things being equal, an environment that is consistently viewed as threatening can certainly contribute to any other individual risk factors for mental health disorders.

---

## Looking Back, Looking Forward

Taking a moment to review the ground we have covered in this chapter, it becomes clear that the ancients were on to something, and that the sanitarium boom, for all the grandiose promises, was surely not a bad thing. If simply viewed in isolation, it might be easy for critics to dismiss some of the research. But when viewed together—when large population studies indicating a stress-buffering effect are layered on top of studies using subjective and objective evaluations of mood and stress, and when this is, in turn, layered onto hospital sickness data and functional brain imaging studies that surely cannot lie—the picture of nature's influence emerges. And when you add on top of that the dozens of shinrin-yoku studies from Japan, with over 1,000 participants and counting, the argument that nature has no consequence on human health and physiology becomes impossible to support.

The brain is absolutely influenced by nature, and it is no longer an option to write off the philosophers and poets as mere romantic dreamers. The results of the scientific investigations reviewed in this chapter should serve as a wake-up call for all of us. The mortality of individuals, nations, and even the planet itself is dependent on the recognition and acceptance that nature is part of us. Our perception of stress, our mental state, our immunity, our happiness, and our resiliency are all chemically influenced by the nervous system and its response to the natural environment.

# 2
## CHAPTER

# Backs to Nature, Sights on Screens: Are We Happy Yet?

*Wilderness is the raw material out of which man has hammered the artifact known as civilization . . . the shallow-minded modern who has lost his rootage in the land assumes that he has already discovered what is important.*

—Professor Aldo Leopold, 1948

Undoubtedly, our technology has served to advance the human animal through all reaches of the planet. Tools have served us well, and just as surely as we have evolved side by side with nature by learning how to seek out sustenance and shelter in the natural environment, we have evolved alongside our tools and technology. The belief that we are capable of bettering ourselves through our own devices is ingrained in us. Our contemporary devices—smartphones, tablets, laptops, and other screen-based gadgets—deliver and provide potentially valuable information; therefore they are in many ways an extension of the tools we have evolved with, and it is easy for us to believe that screen time is nothing but good.

These screen-based gadgets have been sold to us with promises that they'd make our lives easier and better—that we would be filled with happiness in our leisure time, more empathic in our connectivity, and smarter through our instant access to multitudes of information. However, in our brave new technology-rich world, we are more likely to be stressed out, anxious, depressed, distracted, and less inclined to embrace benefit-rich natural environments than ever before. Your authors aren't resistant to technology, and we won't suggest that you should abandon your devices and never set foot in Best Buy again—we won't encourage you to rage against the machine. After all, we humbly appreciate the value of our own gadgets and do find that smartphones can bring order and assistance in times of chaos.

The Internet and its connectivity have countless benefits. From support groups of various types to local and global community organizations, connectivity can be a source of comfort and a mechanism for positive change. Both of us embrace technology and appreciate the many ways in which it has enhanced health care and quality of life. Professionally and personally we rely on computers, use wireless devices and MP3 players, dabble in Facebook—and at least one of us has been known to send a tweet or two. However, we are skeptical of the prevalent sense in Western culture that more technology in our lives and greater immersion in information automatically promotes well-being and happiness. Unfortunately, most of us continue to race to keep up with the latest toys. However, evidence is mounting that chasing technological gadgets for a brighter future—one that never arrives—is taking its toll.

## The False Promise

Almost a half century has passed since virtually every media outlet promised us that computer technology was going to create a massive leisure class. All the experts within the so-called cybernetic revolution were full of glee—computers, these futurists told us, were the panacea for all the individual, social, and global ills. The full-time workweek was going to drop to just 20 hours, and humans would be living a life of near utopia. A 1965 *Time Magazine* cover story told us that "in time the computer will allow man to return to the Hellenic concept of leisure, in which the Greeks had time to cultivate their minds and improve their environment, while slaves did all the labor. The slaves, in modern Hellenism, would be the computer." In a 1967 edition of *Saturday Review*, we were told that "cybernetic slaves produced by the ingenuity of a higher level of man" would usher in a golden age of leisure.

This hasn't quite worked out as planned. In fact, the opposite may be true, as it could easily be argued that many of us have become slaves to our screens. We use the screen to consume some 12 hours of information per day via television, the Internet, texting, music, and games. Researchers who have tracked information consumption since 1980 have found massive increases in info consumption, and it's not just within the workplace: nonwork-related info consumption has increased 350 percent. In 1999, so-called "problem" computer use, the type associated with anxiety and depression, averaged 27 hours a week. Fast-forward to 2012 and we are all way past that average: we could clock 27 hours of screen time in just a few days. We're plowing through information, merely skimming its surface, and we are taking time away from other activities to focus on our screens.

Even if we weren't under the thumb of our devices, we're hardly exploiting our leisure time to our benefit. And, sadly, we can keep dreaming about the 20-hour full-time workweek facilitated by the microchip. What wasn't anticipated was that computers and wireless devices would blur the lines of work and home. Checking work e-mails is standard, even expected, during evenings, weekends, and vacations—75 percent of workers aged 18 to 44 check e-mail while on vacation. And the lure is magnetic: almost 40 percent describe themselves as either frequent or compulsive checkers while on vacation. In the meantime, marketing wizards entice us with the promise that the latest gadget will be *the one*, the *iSomething* that will solve our problems. Never mind that tons of e-devices are considered obsolete and discarded by consumers every year, which should suggest that, in fact, last year's device wasn't *the one*.

Screen culture has not fostered a better world for individuals or, at this point, society. Those who might suggest otherwise will have a difficult time explaining the modern stress epidemic; the high rates of mental health disorders, childhood learning and behavioral disorders, and sleep problems; the declines in IQ; and an overall lack of happiness in regions so chock-full of apps. The "more screens in more places" principle is not promoting health. Marketing continues to sell the notion that the road to happiness is paved with more screens—larger screens for your wall and smaller screens for your pocket—and screen-based social connectivity. Yet, juxtaposed against our social reality, where empathy is down and a trucker is hauling Prozac to a metropolis near you, this is clearly not the case. There is a broad divide between the optimism of cyber-utopia served up in the 1960s and our current state of affairs. A closer examination of North American mental and cognitive health reveals the counterfeit promissory notes written on the technological revolution.

## Stress, Depression, and Anxiety

### Dr. Eva's File

Janet, 43 years old, single and wanting to find love and happiness, knew she had an addiction. With her history of anxiety and post-traumatic stress from childhood trauma, she had built a life for herself that involved work and shopping online. Initially, her addiction to online shopping started innocently. Unable to sleep one night, she perused the information superhighway to keep her mind from spinning. Then she discovered that every time she found a great deal and clicked on the Buy Now button, she experienced a sense of euphoria. The problem now was that she could not stop. Rather than going out socially or meeting people, she chose a date with her on-screen shopping mall. It wasn't so much her loneliness that brought Janet to seek help but the hole in her wallet.

It was a complicated case without a simple solution, but I knew that it was important to figure out a way to get Janet away from the screen and to find new ways to calm her racing mind. When I asked her where her favorite place in nature was, she answered, "The beach. I love the water."

And so, Janet was given two prescriptions: (1) for 10 minutes a day, do guided visualizations involving being near or on the water or beach, especially in the evening when she had difficulty being still, and (2) actually get out to the water or beach.

Over a month's time, Janet started feeling better and more empowered, which motivated her to continue on this path. But she also realized to do so she would require more help, so she joined a support group where she figured she would make friends who would help alleviate some of her loneliness.

Happiness continues to be elusive. For proof, look no further than the 2,000 books with the word "happiness" in the title within amazon.com's Health section—a full 75 percent of all books with the word "happiness" in the title were published after the year 2000. Happiness is loosely defined as having a general satisfaction with life and having more positive than negative emotions (more joy, contentment, vitality, interest, and love; less anger, resentment, guilt, fear, shame, and sadness). Both Canada and the United States are trending down in this category of life satisfaction.

In a 151-country Gallup World Poll, residents of the United States frequently described themselves as sad (68 nations have lower levels of sadness) and angry (74 nations have lower levels of reported anger). Combine this with the epidemic of stress, increasing rates of mental health disorders, and the sheer number of people who sit just below the cutoff for diagnoses of depression and it becomes clear that North American society doesn't exactly ooze happiness. In fact, researchers indicate that less than 20 percent of us are actually flourishing.

Indeed, far from considering themselves happy, the perception of stress among contemporary adults is at an all-time high, which is of great concern, as stress is a driver of physical and mental ill health. North Americans are reporting higher levels of stress and pressure—44 percent say their stress has increased over the last five years. Year by year, the Canadian Mental Health Association reports increasing stress among Canadians. And Americans are a particularly stressed lot, ranking fifth among 151 nations.

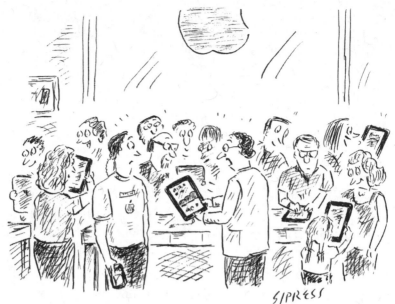

*"I have just one more question—will it make me happy?"*

© David Sipress

The odds of experiencing a mental health disorder are much higher than just a few decades ago. Evaluation of the same personality tests that have been used in U.S. high schools since 1938 indicate that, as of 2007, five times as many students now score above the cutoff for psychopathology. One out of every two North Americans can now anticipate meeting the criteria for a mental health disorder; depression in particular is rampant. Consider that a young adult living in North America today has a 1-in-4 chance of depression, versus 1-in-10 odds of just two generations ago.

Diagnosable mental health disorders, particularly anxiety and depression, typically sit on a continuum. At one end is an adult who is flourishing and content, with mainly positive thoughts and emotions. This individual is not immune to negative thoughts and stressors—no one is—but the scale is simply weighted toward positive emotions. At the other end of the spectrum, a person suffering from anxiety and depression has mainly negative thoughts and is highly reactive to daily hassles and stressors. In reality, more and more individuals are walking wounded, sitting just to the side of diagnosable depression or anxiety. Approximately 30 percent of all visitors to primary care doctors are in this group, regardless of the main complaint. Sitting at this point on the continuum is not benign; it carries with it a compromised quality of life and a diminished mental outlook.

As we write this, huge 18-wheeler trucks are hauling psychotropic medications all over the American interstates and Canadian provincial highways in an effort to help North Americans deal with the fallout from modern life: 12 tons of the four major antianxiety medications annually, 38 tons of the most popular ADHD drug alone, 7 tons of sleeping pills, and 150 tons of antidepressants. Physicians wrote 400 million prescriptions for psychotropic drugs in 2009, four times more than two decades ago, and enough to provide a script for every man, woman, and child in the United States and Canada. Use of these medications and diagnoses of mental health disorders are at an all-time high.

## Diminished Cognitive Edge

Through the 20th century, within developed nations, there was a consistent rise in IQ of about three to five points per decade. Dubbed the Flynn effect (for James Flynn, the researcher who first reported the rising IQ), its wonders have been explained by various factors, including better nutrition, educational improvements, health care, and certain social factors. The factors that have *not* explained the Flynn effect include (but are not limited to) so-called brain-training games, video games, smartphone apps, and other dubious digital training tools. Indeed, it appears the digital-gadget culture may be dumbing us down. Alarm bells have been ringing as researchers show not only a plateau in IQ scores but, even worse, that the Flynn effect is reversing. Large studies from different developed nations have reported a decline in IQ beginning in the late 1990s (in concert with the dawn of digital mania), such that a decade of IQ gains has been wiped out in the years 1998 to 2004.

Even the good Dr. Flynn himself has reported on the reversal: his 2009 study indicated that British teens have experienced an IQ drop from the 1980s' high point. The act of texting and checking e-mail removes 10 available IQ points. Albeit temporary, interruptions of this nature also destroy creativity and lead us down dead ends. For example, a single e-mail interruption will cost a worker an average of 24 minutes from the task at hand. And in the course of a 40-minute study period, a simple texting exchange (less than 3 minutes in duration) will slash a student's word recall in half. We are living in the age of distraction—ADHD rates in children and adults are off the charts.

Although we thought technological advances would make us smarter, evidence is conclusively demonstrating they don't. Consider that:

- Without formally acknowledging that the videos did not create geniuses out of little viewers, Disney has now offered a full refund on any Baby Einstein DVD purchased from 2004 to 2009.
- Researchers have shown that when parents give video-game-naive students (6 to 9 years old) a console, controllers, and rated-E (for "everyone") games, academic performance drops.
- Cognitive psychologist Alain Lieury found that so-called brain-boosting video games actually produce a decline in memorization scores.
- Research involving almost 200 adults showed that teaching older adults to use a computer and navigate the Internet did not improve any aspect of cognitive functioning.

## Decreased Empathy

The digital era was intended to bring us the information superhighway and a means by which to create a force of connectivity—more friends in more places. It has fulfilled these promises, although perhaps not in the way intended. Pioneers did not envision information overload and the way in which information of questionable value can suffocate quality information. Social media were supposed to link us together. Yet, for all the talk of connectivity via gadgets, it does not seem to be translating into a more caring world, at least not in North America. Scores of empathic concern—the ability to exhibit an emotional response to someone else's distress—have dropped 49 percent since 1980. Perspective taking, an intellectual understanding of another person's situational and individual circumstances, has declined by 34 percent.

Heavy Internet users score low on emotional intelligence, which is a measure of how one uses emotions in solving problems. Emotional intelligence is predicated on the ability to use verbal and nonverbal cues to monitor the emotional state of others. This enhances cooperation and understanding in work and social settings, ultimately leading to resiliency to stress and an edge in navigating real-world interactions. In line with lowered emotional intelligence, electrophysiological studies of brain activity have determined that heavy Internet users have alterations in the way they perceive and process the human face. In human interactions, empathy is often predicated on the perception of even the most minor facial cues indicating distress.

The research is clear: when we neglect important social cues in the face of environmental overload, there is, quite simply, a lowered probability of empathy and social concern. The environmental overload can totally remove the conscious perception that others may be in need. Cognitive fatigue can compromise the degree to which one interprets the sometimes subtle cues of need, and the needs of others may be flat-out relegated in importance if they compromise the completion of a multitask. Our devotion to technology and inability to pull ourselves from the screen often comes at the expense of the people around us. For example, a smartphone shuffler (someone texting and walking down a crowded city block) absorbed in the task has a reduced capacity of concern for those in the periphery. This results in a reduced awareness and understanding that by slowly shuffling among harried workers he or she may be invoking pedestrian rage in others. There is no shortage of scientific examples of this, and it doesn't matter whether the broad environment is a relatively small town or a major metropolitan area: an accumulation of distractive environmental inputs to the brain will diminish helpful behavior.

Distractions and information overload in work settings curb the likelihood that the overloaded individual will grant another a favor. The experience of environmental overload leads to impulsivity and results in less time devoted to contemplation, interpretation, and reservation of judgment. Indeed, high environmental overload breeds insensitivity and rapid-fire judgment of others. Judgments made in the presence of environmental overload are reported to be of greater conviction (certainty), and yet they are also more likely to be based on generalizations and less-than-adequate information. Nature immersion, as we will see, is quite the opposite. It restores the brain, buffers the stress of environmental overload, affords opportunity for contemplation, and enhances altruism.

Accompanying this marked drop in concern for and understanding of distress felt by others is a corresponding uptick in self-absorption and narcissism scores. Recent studies have documented significant increases in narcissism among young adults, with 89 percent more students answering almost all personality questions in a narcissistic direction in 2009 compared with 1994. Interestingly, users with the highest scores on narcissistic personality tests are the most frequent daily visitors to Facebook, have more social contacts, and spend the longest time on the site per visit.

Any tilt from empathy to narcissism has enormous consequences for society and the natural environment. Empathy is an essential ingredient in helping behavior and social justice, while the costs of narcissism—exploitation, manipulation, aggression, shallow relationships, and loss of emotional intimacy—are paid for by its victims. Narcissism is also associated with taking undue risk and impulsivity without regard to downstream consequences. Research suggests that collective narcissism clouds ethical goals and squanders resources, encouraging a policy where profiteering is paramount. In a study by a team of psychologists led by W. Keith Campbell, those with the narcissistic view were more likely to cut down a hypothetical forest with greedy intent, forgoing long-term gains and sustainability. Narcissists are no friends of nature.

## Affecting Longevity and Health

Obviously, medical technology has had a dramatically positive influence on life extension, particularly infancy and childhood mortality, and to some degree later in life. Yet, we cannot confuse this wondrous technology and medical advances with the day-to-day gadgets and screens, the devices that surround us under the umbrella term of "technology." When we are stressed and distracted, we often turn to our screens in the hopes they will save us. But the magnetic screen may only serve to increase our risk of dying. Noted cultural critic Neil Postman said it all in the title of his classic book *Amusing Ourselves to Death*. And now, some 30 years later, the research pours in, showing that the screen, with its unlimited pursuits of trivia, superficial distractions, and amusements, is indeed contributing to early mortality. Yes, Postman was right.

In a 2011 study of over 4,500 adults followed for several years, total screen time was associated with a higher risk of death. And the risk increase was not small: it was 52 percent higher versus those with the least screen time. Surprisingly, exercise or lack thereof wasn't the mediating factor. Among those who logged the highest amount of screen time, being physically active reduced their risk of dying from any cause by a mere 4 percent (to 48 percent higher risk of dying!) compared with those who exercised and had the least screen time. Australian researchers report that lifetime TV viewing time is in itself a factor that reduces life expectancy, carrying with it a comparable risk of mortality with that of obesity and physical inactivity. Consider also that when innovative screen restrictors are placed on televisions and computers (shaving off about two hours of screen time per day), the end result is a reduction in body mass index and caloric intake in young children with obesity.

---

### Fear of Free-Range

Research shows that parental fear is one of the driving forces behind kids' leisure-time screen use and indoor recreation. As television, computer, and smartphone news, with its steady diet of horrific crimes and tragedies, gets pumped into their visual cortex, parents perceive the world as a very scary place. Subsequently, indoors seems a far safer place to be. New York City resident Lenore Skenazy, author of the 2009 bestselling *Free-Range Kids*, has started a backlash against this out-of-proportion, media-magnified perception of risk to children in the outdoor world. Sadly, a life of screen confinement is far from safe; it facilitates depression, anxiety, and risk of subsequent psychological difficulties.

---

Overstimulation breeds fatigue in an immediate way by taxing the brain and indirectly by reducing sleep quantity and quality. The sales of caffeinated energy drinks, a $9 billion business in the United States, should be enough to tell us that we are hardly living with an abundance of energy. The intake of caffeine among teens has more than doubled since 1989. For more concrete statistics, we can look to the latest Stress in America survey: 41 percent of American adults are fatigued. Exhaustion is a gaping wound, and energy drinks are only a Band-Aid.

## Wired for Info-Desire

Why can't we tear ourselves away from an excess of information and use it in moderation, when it's clearly taking a toll on us mentally and physically? It's simple, really: at the superficial level, the info-swim feels damn good, and you can blame it all on dopamine. It turns out that we are wired to crave information—big time. To ensure our survival, the brain releases dopamine into its pathways to reward us for finding essentials, such as food and water. New research shows that the brain also uses dopamine to reward information seeking. This seems rational enough; after all, information can be life saving. Yet, there is a dark side to the dopamine reward system in the brain: it can overwhelm other control circuits and elevate the importance of one type of reward at the expense of others. High-calorie food, alcohol, and addictive drugs are examples of the types of rewards that can be elevated in importance and overrun the brain's control systems. We need food for survival, but an abundance of calories in the form of sugar-laden snacks can do great harm if the controls for balance are overridden.

Information, regardless of its quality, is now emerging as a type of highly palatable food in its ability to fire up the dopamine reward neurons. Once the dopamine reward system is engaged, it will in turn further reinforce information seeking. In a sea of instant information and trivia, the info-rewards are numerous and at the ready to fire up the brain's reward system. This explains a lot about why we can't extract ourselves from our gadgets. It explains why taking a tech break is so difficult. Quite simply, that incoming text or unopened e-mail is like a tiny little gift wrapped up with a bow; it's got your name on it, and it might just provide valuable information. And that latest news item on the extracurricular activities of a professional athlete or the marriage of a Hollywood celebrity is like a micro-bowl of delicious hot fudge sundae—so you read it. However, there's never just one e-mail, one text, or one article to read; there are hundreds per day. The days of the odd viral video setting the web abuzz are gone; now there are countless daily viral videos. There is not just one celebrity scandal, there are hundreds, and there are thousands of blogs chronicling them, each with many reader comments for your review.

This global village we have created offers far too many tiny little gifts wrapped up with bows. We are overloaded with information, and we struggle to separate information of actual value to us from that which is akin to junk food. The fast-food-style info merely provides a temporary feel-good fix in the form of a little jolt of dopamine in the reward centers of the brain. Thoreau didn't know about dopamine's powerful pull, but he was aware that people tend to have an attraction to information of dubious quality. In *Walden* he writes, "We are in great haste to construct a magnetic telegraph from Maine to Texas; but Maine and Texas, it may be, have nothing important to communicate . . . we are eager to tunnel under the Atlantic and bring the Old World some weeks nearer to the New; but perchance the first news that will leak through into the broad flapping American ear will be that Princess Adelaide has the whooping cough."

Although not official diagnoses yet, "Internet addiction" and "digital-device addiction" are terms batted around by the medical community. Currently, 42 percent of Americans flat-out agree with the statement that they "cannot live without" their mobile phone, and more than half of adults also state that both they and their kids spend too much time online. Although estimates vary, it seems that some 10 percent of the population qualifies as having a full-blown Internet addiction. The obvious reason for not being able to unplug and power down is the fear of missing something. In truth, we're already missing something—sleep, face-to-face interaction, contemplation time, physical activity, and a little immersion in the natural environment, to name just a few things. But at least we now have a credible defense for being hypnotized by our devices: "Dopamine made me do it!"

## Daily Hassles and Stress Physiology

> *If you ask what is the single most important key to longevity, I would have to say it is avoiding worry, stress and tension. And if you didn't ask me, I'd still have to say it.*
> —George F. Burns

## Dr. Eva's File

Fred sat in my office looking for help with stress management. It wasn't his idea; it was his wife's. She had threatened to leave him if he didn't seek help. During the one-hour visit, Fred checked his incoming text messages five times and answered two of the four phone calls, saying first, "Do you mind? This is important."

From the history I was able to get, it turned out Fred, who had an "important" job, spent 12 hours a day working, including during his hour-long daily commute, allowing little time for exercise, self-care, or downtime.

I asked him, "What do you think you would have done if you were in this office 20 years ago when smartphones, e-mail, and such did not exist?" He thought for a minute before answering, "Probably pay attention and learn how to relax."

I then explained to Fred the consequences of an overactivated stress response system that does not have the chance to get a break, rest, or relax: depression and anxiety, heart disease and hypertension, inflammatory disorders, musculoskeletal problems, memory loss, immune compromise (making one more susceptible to infection) . . . "Shall I continue?" I asked.

Much has been written on the influence of stress in human health. Early on, this research focused on the connection between major stressors—significant life changes, major losses, and trauma—and their detrimental effects on physical and mental well-being. More recently, researchers have been looking closely at the health-erosive properties of chronic low-grade stress. Like waves eroding a shoreline, a steady stream of minor stressors can also take a toll on health and well-being. Traffic, noise, quarrels at home and work, disagreements with neighbors, encounters with incivility, and locking horns with customer service departments are just some examples of what psychologists term "daily hassles." These hassles are technically defined as events, thoughts, or situations that produce negative feelings such as annoyance, agitation, anxiety, frustration, worry, or a general sense of irritation. Hassles are usually perceived as roadblocks to meeting specific goals. With this definition in mind, it is easy to see how the digital age has added a new dimension—a slow-walking smartphone shuffler might make you late for a meeting, or a loud cell-phone talker in your vicinity might distract you as you're trying to finish writing a report. These, plus many other modern intrusions, contribute to an average of 50 brief stress response episodes per day for North American adults.

These daily hassles are far from benign. They are now emerging as even better predictors of depression onset and recurrence than are major life stressors. The emotional response to a hassle sets off a cascade of stress physiology, including an uptick in production of the stress hormone cortisol. Otherwise healthy adults who report high work stress have high cortisol levels, as do adults suffering from anxiety and depression. In general, workers who report excess commitments, time constraints in the face of daily assignments, and postponement of recreation due to workload have significantly higher cortisol levels than their less-stressed counterparts. Associations between anger and higher cortisol levels among employees have also been noted. Although cortisol has some short-term health advantages during a legitimate crisis (for example, immune support), long-term elevations via environmental overload are destructive. In particular, chronic cortisol elevations are associated with a cycle of low-grade inflammation and oxidative stress, which can damage cells. The venomous tandem of chronic inflammation and oxidative stress has been linked to virtually every chronic medical condition, from acne to ulcers. Worse still is that cortisol elevations, inflammation, and oxidative stress, once thought to be a mere consequence of anxiety and depression, appear to play a causative role in further amplifying mood disturbances. The entire cascade may directly assault nerve cells and lower the availability of mood-regulating neurotransmitters.

The cascade of health-compromising chemicals prompted by stress can change your entire worldview. Cortisol, when administered to healthy adults, can diminish the normal level of brain arousal when these subjects are shown the image of a happy face.

When a depressed mood state is induced in otherwise healthy adults, the world becomes a more painful place, both physically (pain perception is amplified) and emotionally. When levels of inflammatory chemicals are intentionally elevated in content, normal adults under experimental settings, they cause changes in mental outlook, including increases in anxious feelings, depressive thoughts, and cognitive brain fog.

Daily hassles also turn us away from healthy behaviors. For example, daily hassles are associated with an increased consumption of high-fat and sugary snacks and a simultaneous increase in the likelihood of skipping meals and avoiding vegetables. Suffice it to say that under the influence of daily hassles we are not reaching for broccoli and Swiss chard. It has also been noted that those who report a high incidence of daily hassles are less likely to engage in intentional physical activity. This is reflected in recent Stress in America surveys, with about 40 percent of respondents stating that they deal with stress by turning on the television and an additional 35 percent stating that they go to another screen (computer, video gaming) for solace. This shouldn't be surprising because under stress we need that hit of dopamine more than ever. Sophisticated brain imaging studies have shown that stress itself causes changes in brain activity that amplify a voracious desire to return to the object of our cravings.

What the brain really needs in the face of daily hassles is a shot of positive emotion. Just as surely as hassles can provoke the cascade of stress, daily uplifts can cut it off. Increased uplifting experiences are independently associated with a reduction in inflammation. "Independently" is the key word: it tells us that we can make positive emotions work for us even in the face of the daily hassles. Put another way, induction of positive emotions can trump hassles. Indeed, researchers have shown that when it comes to a head-to-head face-off, it is the absence of positive emotions (versus the presence of negative emotions) that more accurately predicts ill health and even mortality.

### Canaries in the Coal Mine

> Once I was let down into a deep well into which choke-damp had settled, and nearly lost my life. The deeper I was immersed in the invisible poison, the less capable I became of willing measures of escape from it. And in just this condition are those who toil or dawdle or dissipate in crowded towns, in the sinks of commerce or pleasure.
>
> —John Muir

The age of the screen is relatively new, and the long-term impact of excessive exposure to information has been undocumented until recently. Studies looking at those who are immersed in screen culture—whose Internet-based lives may foreshadow what's in store for the culture at large—are starting to roll in, and the results do not bode well for these canaries in the coal mine, nor do they bode well for the rest of us. These studies have examined what happens when physically and mentally healthy youth and young adults record screen time and are tracked over time. When followed over two to seven years, the screen media consumption, video game use, and computer use at the beginning of the study was associated with an increased risk that these otherwise healthy youths and adults would subsequently experience depression, anxiety (particularly social anxiety), psychological difficulties, and less sleep.

When a large group of over 4,100 nondepressed teens are followed for seven years, and screen media consumption predicts later depression in young adulthood, we must surely rethink everything. Research clearly shows that exposure to violent video games predicts an increase in aggression and a dip in empathy. Now that we know significant immersion in any sort of video games predicts anxiety and depression, it is time to sit up and take notice.

## Screen Culture and Nature Displacement

*If future generations are to remember us with
gratitude rather than contempt, we must leave them
more than the miracles of technology. We must
leave them a glimpse of the world as it was in the
beginning, not just after we got through with it.*

—Lyndon Johnson

U.S. President Johnson made the comment quoted above as he signed the 1964 Wilderness Act, presuming that the miracles of technology would not dampen the desire to glimpse unspoilt nature. However, in 1964, even the best of futurists could not predict the extent to which the screen would change the brain and our relationship to each other and the natural world. Researchers have suggested that in a world filled with screen-based stimulation and hyperreality, nature might not be exciting enough; indeed, it might be boring. Certainly, there are troubling signs that nature is losing its appeal and that the desire to get a mindful glimpse of its wonders is waning. The LED screens, video game controllers, and so-called man caves are becoming far too attractive to abandon for the woods.

A recent study in the *Proceedings of the National Academy of Sciences* indicates that overall nature-based recreation has decreased 50 percent in the last four decades. The expansion of daily screen time is coinciding with a broad nature displacement effect. According to University of Illinois scientist Oliver Pergams and colleague Patricia Zaradic, our entire society appears to be making a "pervasive shift away from nature-based recreation." These researchers have identified indoor entertainment and screens—home and commercial theater, computer use, television viewing time, video games—as associated variables in the shift away from visits to national parks.

Although it is difficult to prove definitively that screens have displaced visitation to national, state, and provincial parks, there are only so many hours in a day, and given that total daily consumption of entertainment media has increased dramatically, it remains a viable argument. Today, children and teens consume an unfathomable 7 hours and 38 minutes per day engaged with media outside school. In 1988, when national park visits started on their current downward trend, declining as much as 25 percent, the average time spent playing home-video games and surfing the Internet was negligible. In 1999, those aged 8 to 18 spent 26 minutes a day playing video games and 27 minutes on a computer outside school; today, these numbers are 1 hour 13 minutes and 1 hour 29 minutes respectfully, with an extra 42 minutes of daily TV viewing thrown on top compared with 1999. Visits to U.S. state parks have also declined in the last two decades. Their high point was recorded in 1990—the same year the Nintendo World Championships competition toured 30 American cities and fanned the flames of home and portable video game culture. Parks Canada reported a 6 percent reduction in visits to Canadian national parks and national historic sites from 2004 to 2009. Minnesota, a state known for some of the most impressive outdoor recreation opportunities, has witnessed a dramatic drop in nature-based recreation since 1996. Use of the famous Boundary Waters Canoe Area Wilderness (BWCA), with its million acres of wilderness and over 1,000 pristine lakes and streams, has dropped almost 30 percent among residents since 1996. Could it have something to do with the fact that the BWCA is outside the tech world and, at least as we write, one of the few remaining areas in North America without a mobile phone tower?

The ascent of screen culture has occurred in association with the decline in mindful engagement with nature. The benefits of being in green are being obscured by the powerful pull of the dopamine reward system and the information vortex. There is a personal loss here: we are becoming less aware of the mentally rejuvenating and cognitively restorative benefits of nature. There is also an environmental loss: a collective detachment is not in the interest of conservation. Although there is much talk about environmental awareness and "being green," when it comes to being green in the true sense—connecting with nature and actually being *in* green in a mindful sense—our society is losing its way. Screen-based gadgets are luring us away from nature and all its benefits. It's not possible to cultivate true concern and empathy for nature while being completely detached from it. True connectivity in any relationship, be it interpersonal or with elements of nature, serves to strengthen empathy and concern. Mostly, we stand up for what we know and what we have experienced. Yet, at a time when we need conservation efforts more than ever, when we need a little stress relief more than ever, we are turning our backs on nature.

## The Fork in the Road—What Are We Losing and What Can We Gain?

> *I went to the woods because I wished to live*
> *deliberately, to front only the essential facts of life,*
> *and see if I could not learn what it had to teach, and*
> *not, when I came to die, discover that I had not lived.*
>
> —Henry David Thoreau

It has been said that Thoreau's retreat to solitude and nature immersion was a backtrack to a fork in the road, to a place where humans had veered off course in a misguided search for wisdom and happiness. Obviously, that fork does not exist on any archived Rand McNally atlas and in the age of high technology, any contemporary back-to-nature search for it would be as pointless as seeking out the location of Ponce de Leon's Fountain of Youth. Moving past the romanticized notions of life in the woods, we can certainly learn from what was once there at that fork. We can look to the anthropological evidence and screen-less hunter-gatherer communities to obtain information about the brain as it was once on nature. Cross-cultural studies certainly indicate that a traditional way of life is protective against depression, while on the other hand, the degree of modernization is indeed associated with increased rates of depression.

Clearly, we do not need to return to a hunter-gatherer lifestyle or live in Thoreau's cabin to avoid screens and cities—we simply need to examine the benefits of what is disappearing. In the pages that follow, we explore scientific studies and share direct clinical experiences that make it abundantly clear that nature should not be forgotten. Rather than poetic and romantic tales of nature, it is science that is now showing us there is indeed a downside when the technological pendulum swings too far away from the natural world. It has become clear that we have hurtled toward yet another major junction in our evolution—the yellow cautionary road sign is in sight, and a decision must be made. What will our societal GPS tell us to do? Will we recalculate? Will we learn to strike a good balance of technology and nature, or will we continue becoming part of the machine? We don't have to go back to Thoreau's fork; we need to be mindful of the one right in front of us.

To fully appreciate the new fork at which we have found ourselves, consider a 2009 study published in *Personality and Social Psychology Bulletin*. Researchers at the University of Rochester examined the effects of nature immersion on life aspirations. There are two general categories of life aspirations, intrinsic and extrinsic, both of which can influence important decisions, judgments, perceptions, and overall direction in life. Extrinsic aspirations are focused on goods, such as fame, money, and image. Intrinsic aspirations are those that support basic psychological needs, including personal growth, community, and intimacy. In short, intrinsic aspirations involve values that might be described as prosocial. In the study, participants viewed four photographic images of natural environments (and separately, human-made city scenes) and were asked to imagine themselves fully immersed in the environments (considering the potential sounds, smells, colors, textures) for about eight minutes. After this procedure, the subjects answered a series of questions designed to evaluate the degree to which they were psychologically immersed in the environment, as well as any effects on aspirations and altruism. Viewing the human-made city scenes predicted a higher value of extrinsic aspirations; it seems that the city view jacks up the desire for money, power, and fame—the self is prioritized. Those who viewed the city scenes were also less likely to share resources with others. This finding is, perhaps, unsurprising. Maybe viewing a cityscape provokes thoughts of money, fame, and fortune because it taps into our cultural learning; maybe we are simply socialized to perceive the city as an every-man-and-woman-for-themselves environment. In contrast, those who viewed the nature scenes and felt truly immersed in nature placed a much higher value on intrinsic aspirations. In fact, these scenes produced an attitudinal shift such that the participants were more concerned with prosocial goals than they were before being immersed in nature, and they were also more willing to give to others.

The investigators then moved away from the photographic images. This time they had a separate group of 75 young adults complete similar tests of aspirations and evaluate how they would divvy up money as they sat in one of two rooms, identical except for one feature: the presence or absence of vegetation. Specifically, one room had two floor plants, one potted plant on a corner table, and one on the desk where the surveys were completed. Incredibly, the mere presence of four plants in a room produced a robust and significant elevation of intrinsic aspirations. Further, the presence of natural vegetation mediated higher scores on feeling connected to nature and subsequent generosity compared with those who took the very same tests in a room without plants. This is a bit harder to explain than simply cultural learning; it indicates that something deeper is going on, something underappreciated in our technoculture, that is, that the loss of 2 million years of evolutionary nature contact may be damaging true connectivity to each other and to our planet.

In the context of this totality of time spent in evolutionary contact with nature, modern technology has brought about rapid environmental changes. As isolated groups of scientists grapple in their efforts to determine how screen culture is changing the brain, and separate groups examine nature's untold influence, it is becoming clear that these are not distinct discussions. Too often, our immersion in the digital world is viewed in isolation, without consideration for what is being lost by the corresponding shift from the natural environment. Researchers mostly focus on how the Internet or screen devices change aspects of brain information processing or interpersonal communication. However, an equally important and contextual construct relates to how the Internet/screen world and nature deprivation are combining to synergistically change the human brain and behavior. Modern science is validating Thoreau's feelings that "we can never have enough of nature" and that in nature "is the preservation of the world." Wilson's biophilia hypothesis seems to be correct, and yet, we humans are wrenching ourselves further away from nurturing nature. As the remaining chapters unfold, it will become clear that the broad aspects of nature, as well as some of its specific elements, can influence the human brain and brain-directed aspects of health.

# 3

# Nature and Cognition: What Can Green Do for You?

*I doubt whether artificial stimulants ever promote*
*growth either of body or mind. They may increase*
*power for a single effort, but that power is drawn*
*from the system, not imparted to it, and must leave*
*the energies of the system reduced and prostrated.*
*Instead, then, of increasing, it has reduced its capital*
*stock of power.*

—William W. Mitchell, editor, *Massachusetts Teacher,* 1852

In late 2008, the Internet was alight with blazing headlines: neuroscientists had discovered that Google was "making us smarter" and "improving the mind." Too bad neuroscientists hadn't discovered anything of the sort. What the researchers had actually shown was that older adults with a greater history of Internet use—compared with so-called Net-naive adults—had increased arousal in a wide variety of brain regions while performing an Internet search task. Contrary to the media hype, arousal in the brain does not simply equate to smartness. Any individual with an Internet addiction, drug addiction, or craving will also exhibit widely increased brain signal intensity when they see even extremely remote cues related to what they are drawn to—this does not mean they are smarter!

Unfortunately, popular culture perceives arousal as being synonymous with focus and intelligence. Consequently, we consume a steady diet of more stimulation, more energy drinks, more video games, more caffeine, more sugar—basically, more everything. Unquestionably, arousal in the brain and stimulation in response to mental challenges, especially to novel material, is a means of supporting the growth and protection of our nerve cells—to a point. There is no argument from us that the use-it-or-lose-it philosophy to cognitive fitness is correct, and we readily acknowledge that arousal and stimulation strengthen cognitive performance. However, there is also a flip side to the brain fitness story beyond that of puzzles and games, one that is equally important and yet consistently overlooked.

Rarely does the contemporary brain-boosting story take into consideration the real-world cost of a little cognitive something called inhibition fatigue. Inhibition is a crucial brain regulatory function, the orchestra conductor of cognitive function that diverts brain energy stores away from distractions and toward important attentional tasks. In the modern world, with its multitude of distractions, the filtering systems need to work overtime to keep dampening down the influence of information excess. For example, in the screen-based world, the brain must work hard to eliminate the features of web pages that are of little relevance to the information that is being sought—toolbars, pop-ups, advertisements, irrelevant linked articles to the left and right of the main text.

In addition to working harder in the face of ever-present distractions, the modern brain must also contend with an increasing number of routine decisions, thanks to very broad consumer choice. The overwhelming amount of choice we have in contemporary society calls for a tremendous amount of energy to run the pathways of executive functioning in the brain. These areas are involved in planning, abstract thinking, creativity, and so-called cognitive flexibility, and very importantly, they are the centers that involve self-control. As a microcosm of choice, consider that in 1976 there were some 9,000 different items in North American supermarkets; today we have more than 40,000 unique items in an average-sized super-market. Consider also the 100-plus channels available to the average cable TV–consuming household—so many channels, what to watch? Research shows that we use up mental energy when faced with multiple options, and that the energy depletion is more pronounced in the areas of the brain that control our unhealthy cravings, so self-control diminishes—think overeating, overspending, and indulging in impulsive, risky behavior. The toll for the greater demand for inhibition in the brain is an expensive one, and it will ultimately be paid in the form of inhibition fatigue. Researchers now commonly refer to this condition as directed attention fatigue.

## The Discovery of Directed Attention Fatigue

Writing in the late 1800s, Harvard psychologist William James pondered why many office workers experienced mental fatigue. He noted a distinction between two major forms of attention: that which required sustained effort (voluntary attention) and an effortless process (involuntary attention) wherein there was a degree of interest or excitement. Think of voluntary attention as work, a form of mental volunteerism—it's like raising your hand and purposefully agreeing to an assignment for which you must hold your attention to cognitive tasks—say, for example, extracting various bits of information from Excel files before the mid-morning coffee break. With involuntary attention there is no volunteering, no raising of the hand to say, "Okay, I'll do it," no purposeful agreement; it's not really work at all—it simply happens without effort.

James perceived that office workers, those contending with drudging detail and uninteresting interactions, would be continually faced with the daunting task of trying to maintain voluntary attention. He proposed that prolonged voluntary attention would take its toll in the form of what he termed "the uncomfortable feeling of strain." In short, prolonged periods of focused attention require a tremendous amount of effort. Trying to mentally shake oneself back into a state of voluntary attention with "pulses of effort" was a problem in the making. "In all respects, reliance upon such attention as this is a wasteful method, bringing bad temper, and nervous wear and tear as well as imperfect results," the psychologist wrote. On the other hand, those who could exceed in the cognitive realm were able to take advantage of greater immersion in the mode of involuntary attention; they made continuous and interesting associations between thoughts or, as James called it, a thought pattern that "once started, develops all sorts of fascinating consequences." The protection against cognitive fatigue was being supported by fascination, and it would be easier to stay on task with energy if the subject matter was of interest. Geniuses, as James referred to cognitively fit people, were being sustained on passive or involuntary attention, such that cognitive effort wasn't really effort at all.

James's contemporaries expanded on his work, speaking of the debilitating mental fatigue induced by extended periods of voluntary attention. Psychologist Edward Thorndike, a student of James, pointed out that it is not the work expended in the administrative details of an office setting or the algebra in a schoolhouse per se that causes mental fatigue; it is the high energy cost of "inhibiting the tendencies to think of other things." In other words, mental fatigue was being amplified by firing up the areas of the brain that are required to put the brakes on distracting thoughts. It is sort of like driving a car while also applying some pressure to the brake pedal—it is not incredibly efficient. On the one hand, when we are immersed in an environment where stimuli (objects) are naturally attractive to us, Thorndike maintained, "it wins place over other thoughts without any feeling of effort on our part." If the task at hand (or stimuli) "is attractive and absorbing, fatigue diminishes."

James's contemporaries understood that as distractions pile up, the amount of effort required to stay on task increases, and so does the rate of mental fatigue. In particular, the focus on promoting involuntary attention, a form of attention that they aptly referred to as "primitive," was thought to be of critical value to those with mental health disorders. Max E. Witte, a psychiatrist in Iowa, proposed that work "on the farm and in the garden should be more extensively employed for the betterment of these people" because it promotes attention "of the involuntary type." His position was that tipping the scale toward involuntary attention "lessens the disturbances and wear on the individual." As the superintendent of Iowa's primary hospital for mental health, Clarinda State, Witte stated in 1899 that when it comes to the promotion of involuntary attention through activities, "the great majority can find it only by delving in the soil." Witte reported that his own observations among thousands of patients made it clear that physical contact with nature has a profoundly beneficial influence on mental processes, a benefit that most often goes unnoticed and unattributed to the nature contact. This century-old research certainly provides a clear reason as to why the brain is working attentional overtime while it is "on Google," and it opened the doors to understanding how involuntary attention can influence your cognitive brain on nature. Still, it was, in the eyes of a world leaning toward science and evidence only, merely observational and anecdotal. It would take the better part of a century before scientists would start to try to connect the dots between James and the contention that delving in the soil might provide a cognitive advantage.

## Attention Restoration Theory

In 1977, psychologist Dr. Stephen Kaplan advanced the work of James and his peers by establishing a working hypothesis in that nature itself might provide cognitive restoration via its ability to take the load off all the inhibitory effort required in our modern world. Kaplan posited that natural environments are fascinating environments and, as such, they hold involuntary attention without requiring the expenditure of energy in the brain that would otherwise cause cognitive fatigue. Nature experiences have the ability to promote a sense of cognitive clarity wherein there is an absence of confusion. This type of mental focus has served humans well in the natural environment for millions of years. As Kaplan noted, being in a state of mental fatigue, lost in distracting thoughts, would have been quickly fatal on the African savanna. The fascination afforded by natural environments ensured our survival by promoting mental clarity without requiring great amounts of energy. However, in modern society, the bulk of our experiences have minimal intrinsic fascination and, as Kaplan said, "the interesting is no longer important." In other words, all of the modern-day infotoxins (the information of dubious quality) lure us in under the guise of interest, but because they are not important and do not hold fascination, they tend to become an energy sink.

Although directed attention fatigue is a temporary state, one that can be reset with some uninterrupted and distraction-free downtime, survival in the modern urban savanna requires a fair amount of voluntary attention, so we prop ourselves up with caffeine, energy drinks, supplements, drugs, and amusements. Kaplan hypothesized that the mental fatigue induced by applying the brakes in the brain as it accelerates through the nonfascinating demands of the modern world could be remedied by environmental settings that are involuntarily fascinating, effortlessly engaging the inhabitants. Kaplan said, "If nature could be shown to have this property, then the popularity of natural settings for recovery from overload and stress would make considerable sense." The legitimate cognitive energy drink might be in the form of a forest bath.

Kaplan formalized the initial cognitive-nature theory as the attention restoration theory (ART), with four major components proposed for the cognitively restorative environment:

1. **Being away**: while being away can be viewed as getting away from the routine drudgery in the physical or geographic sense, it need not be a physical removal from the source of voluntary attention. Being away may be as simple as mentally reframing the current environment or changing the direction of the visual field. Being away can simply be closing one's eyes and visualizing nature, or shifting focus off the Excel files and looking out a window to a view of nature.

2. **Fascination**: humans are clearly fascinated by the natural world. From ladybugs and centipedes to rounded stones on a

creek bed and driftwood, from sand dunes to snow banks, from bonsai to giant sequoias, it can clearly hold our attention. The distinction in ART is the experience of "soft" fascination (such as viewing a sunset) as a means to cognitive restoration versus "hard" fascination (such as attending an NHL game). While both might be fascinating and capable of holding involuntary attention, one of these, the sunset, affords greater opportunity for cognitive refreshment.

3. **Extent**: the environment must have a considerable depth such that it engages the mind to a significant degree. In the context of ART, a single potted plant probably wouldn't suffice as fitting the criteria for extent, while a field of flowers or a forest would provide ample extent. However, even small urban spaces can provide extent if they use design techniques that magnify the scope of the view (such as a Japanese garden). Further, photographic images of expansive nature scenes can provide visual extent.

4. **Compatibility**: the environment provides a means of fulfilling the individual's activities and intentions without struggle and effort. Most natural environments easily fulfill the criteria of compatibility because they most often fulfill visitors' expectations. From a brief mental respite in a small urban park to a full-fledged recreational experience, humans are generally not disappointed with the outcome upon leaving natural settings.

Kaplan proposed that we might be able to negate the modern dilemma of directed attention fatigue by taking advantage of natural settings. Since most natural settings provide fascination and get your mental view 180 degrees away from the suffocation of Excel files, PowerPoint presentations, and countless activities of voluntary attention, immersion in nature can act as a low-cost brain booster. In the years since Kaplan proposed his theory, a number of studies have supported the cognitive benefits of attention restoration via natural settings. In a 2005 study, researchers induced mental fatigue in their subjects through a cognitively demanding task, one that required the effort of voluntary attention. After the subjects were mentally fatigued, the researchers presented them with photographic images that were previously evaluated for restoration potential. Half of the group viewed images that had been reported to be high in restoration potential—scenes that were, not surprisingly, of forests, water, mountains, beaches, and so on. The other half of the mentally fatigued group viewed low-restoration pictures, such as scenes of city streets with multiple cars, industrial zones, housing developments, and factories. After viewing some 25 photographs of either high or low restorative potential for five minutes, the subjects delved back into the same cognitively demanding task for another five minutes. The group who viewed the restorative nature scenes had better results than those who viewed the urban scenes—demonstrating higher sensitivity in detecting the target as requested, faster reaction time, and a higher number of correct responses to the challenge. The same research group has recently replicated the findings of improved reaction time (after induced mental fatigue and rechallenge with a cognitive test) after viewing nature scenes rated high in fascination. They also reported overall better memory recall after viewing scenes of nature compared with built urban scenes.

### Urban Forest as Brain Booster

In a 2011 study, researchers in Seoul, South Korea, a city fortunate enough to have an immense urban national park system, set up an experiment to evaluate the cognitive effects of a walk through a pine forest versus downtown streets. The subjects completed cognitive and mood tests up front and proceeded on their 50-minute walks. After the walks, the participants were subjected to further cognitive testing. At a later date, the groups were switched: the urban walkers took the forest walk and vice versa. The results showed the expected elevations in mood among the forest walkers compared with the urban walkers, and they also revealed that only after the forest walks did participants score improvements in cognition.

Further support of the original ART comes from an elegant 2008 study published in *Psychological Science*. Researchers induced mental fatigue with a series of challenging brain games designed to put pressure on voluntary attention. Immediately following a 35-minute period of intense experimental cognitive brain drain and testing, the subjects took a walk either in a lush park or on city streets. After the walk, the cognitive tests were repeated and once again the results showed a significant performance difference in favor of those who had spent time in nature. In a separate portion of the same study, researchers also confirmed that viewing photographic nature scenes improved scores of executive attention, which involves management of short-term memory and is essential for minimizing the interference of distracting side shows while on task. In this study, the subjects experienced cognitive refreshment without changes in their mood per se. In other words, we cannot write off these mental gains provided by nature as simply an artifact of less anxiety and a more positive outlook. This finding points to a direct cognitive replenishment through nature experience. It suggests that beyond all the benefits to mood, nature also has the distinct ability to allow us to drive cognitively without applying the brakes. Nature, without wearing down the brake pads of inhibition (fascination and decreased demand for inhibitory energy), minimizes the directed attention fatigue. This, of course, does not mean that ART is not of relevance to those with anxiety, depression, and high levels of daily stress—it most certainly is, particularly because cognitive restoration is an important factor in keeping subsequent stress at bay. Someone may walk through an urban park, or spend time within it, not necessarily noting any significant change in mood, yet he or she is better equipped for the next big cognitive hurdle.

## Why Cognitive Restoration Matters

In the urban world, as work has shifted away from technologically unassisted physical labor, success often depends on voluntary attention to cognitively demanding tasks. While looking for valuable information within documents, files, web pages, texts, tweets, and instant messages, and at the same time blocking out pop-up ads, toolbars, side stories, irrelevant yet tempting must-see YouTube sensations, we are again driving with one foot on the accelerator and the other on the brake. Cognitive fatigue sets in fast. It doesn't matter if you are in a corporate cubicle with your eye on the brightly lit corner office or a student trying to fulfill your potential; if you want to stay ahead of the pack, you must not let mental fatigue drag you down.

If the mentally fatigued brain is left without proper refreshment, the results are not pretty. In recent years, various studies have shown that mental fatigue diminishes our ability to ignore irrelevant information, magnifies the unimportant, and makes us absolutely more prone to distraction. Not only do mentally fatigued subjects make more errors but they cannot recognize mistakes that they would easily pick up on if they were in an optimal zone of mental performance. In addition, mental fatigue decreases our ability to plan ahead and to be flexible with our thoughts. Mental fatigue diminishes the view of the details, so-called local processing. You might see the house, but you cannot see the bricks and mortar. In a mentally fatigued state, people can maintain thoughts and behaviors that run on autopilot, but if something out of the norm were to happen, they would be in a bad spot because they'd be less capable of dealing with the novel situation and information.

Mental fatigue is also fully capable of impairing physical performance in healthy adults. Consider a 2009 study published in the *Journal of Applied Physiology* where subjects performed cognitively demanding computer tests and then jumped on a stationary bike. The control group also exercised on the bike, except they had just watched an emotionally neutral documentary on the *Orient Express* or Ferrari (the nature content of these videos was not reported). The differences between the groups on the cycle-to-exhaustion test were remarkable: the mentally fatigued group gave up quickly, having reached a maximal level of perceived exertion much faster, and reported their perception of effort to be significantly higher during the exercise than their counterparts in the control group. In short, the mentally fatigued mind causes a tired body. Obviously, this provides an explanation as to why it is so difficult for many mentally overworked adults to get out and exercise.

William James described a feeling of strain that built up in association with higher levels of voluntary cognitive demands. This uncomfortable feeling might be an adaptive mechanism, a warning sign to let us know that we are crossing a line into health risk. When strain builds up, we have essentially purchased a ticket to cognitive deficits and diminished performance—that much is clear. Studies of overworked medical residents show that burning the flame of cognitive attention for too long sets the stage for anger and impulsivity. The ultimate destination of unattended mental fatigue is the land of burnout, anxiety, depression, and compromised health. By the same token, chronic stress, anxiety, anger, and depression cause an individual to be much more vulnerable to mental fatigue. Those with anxiety, depression, or both are well known to have deficits in attention, memory, information processing, and executive control. The entire process linking fatigue states and anxiety or depression is a two-way street, and the buffer zone between high cognitive demands and that feeling of strain becomes much smaller when one is chronically stressed.

Adult memory performance can be disturbed by just a few days of elevated levels of the stress hormone cortisol, and even low-level elevation of pro-inflammatory immune chemicals (cytokines) impairs verbal and nonverbal memory. Nature can lower stress hormones and keep inflammation in check, so it follows that nature can be of enormous importance to cognitive health. In sum, it seems that nature can improve cognition by mechanisms involving mood and stress, and also distinctly through taking the weight off voluntary attention and inhibitory demands. But despite this winning, low-cost intervention, in a world full of cognitive demands, many are turning their backs on the restorative powers of nature and reaching instead for another energy drink.

## Academics and Attention Deficit Disorder

> *Lead your child out into Nature. Tutor him on the*
> *hilltop and in the valley. There he will listen better,*
> *and the sense of freedom will give him more strength*
> *to overcome difficulties."*
> —Johann H. Pestalozzi, 1774

In an interesting study published in the *Journal of Environmental Psychology* in 1995, researchers visited the campus dorm rooms of volunteer undergrad students. They placed a Quiet Please sign on the doors and took the students' phones off the hook. Then they performed a series of objective neurocognitive tests of attention. The students were evenly matched in age and academic background, and there was only one major difference in the dorm room environment: the view from the window. One group had a view to nature (trees, lake), a second group had a view of some small amounts of nature but mostly bricks and mortar, and a third group had a view of a completely human-built environment (bricks, slate rooftops). Those with the unobstructed view of nature outperformed their peers on the objective measures of attention. They also reported higher subjective perceptions of attention than those with obstructed or non-natural views.

In a study published in 2010, Dr. Rodney H. Matsuoka of the University of Michigan set out to evaluate the relationship between classroom views to nature and academic performance. The study involved 101 public high schools in Michigan, and in addition to scaling classroom views for the degree and types of nature, there were evaluations of the window views from the primary cafeteria of each school. Even after controlling for socioeconomic factors, class size, age of the school facilities, and other factors, the results showed that classroom and cafeteria views to green vegetation were significant factors in academic performance on standardized tests. Moreover, views to trees and shrubs were associated with higher graduation rates and future plans for attendance at four-year university programs. "Trees" and "shrubs" are key words because the degree of naturalness within the view mattered—a view to mowed grass was not a promoter of academic performance. Separate research involving analysis of 71 rural and suburban elementary schools (data representing over 10,000 fifth-grade students) showed that a view to the outside world of green and the living—not parking lots and walls—was associated with higher scores on reading, language proficiency, and math. Studies also showed that the outdoor classroom, once in vogue in the early 20th century, improves math and science scores compared with instruction in the traditional schoolhouse.

The ability of natural views and settings to influence neurocognitive scores of healthy students led scientists to wonder what the implications might be for those who desperately need support of attentional processes. In 2004, researchers at the University of Illinois caused a stir when they reported that activities conducted in greenspace are associated with symptom reduction of attention deficit/hyperactivity disorder (ADHD) compared with the same activities conducted in built environments. The researchers, using data from 452 parents of children who had been formally diagnosed with ADHD, set out to determine if the setting of some 50 activities (from reading to playing sports) would make a difference in attention. Regardless of age, the presence or absence of hyperactivity in the child, economic bracket, geographic location within the United States, and rural or urban residence, activities in the green outdoors appeared to prove advantageous in reducing symptoms of attention deficit. This was the second time this group of researchers had made such connections—in a previous study involving a smaller sample (96 parents), they had also found that the greenness of play areas was associated with milder symptoms of attention deficit and that windowless indoor play areas were associated with more severe symptoms.

More recently, investigators have performed objective testing of attention in children with ADHD after time spent in natural or built environments. In a European study, researchers conducted a test of concentration after children had engaged in a period of light to moderate physical activity in a natural wooded area or a built town area. The results showed that performance on concentration tasks was higher in those who had played in the wooded environment. The researchers concluded that the concentration and behavior was largely held constant among those in the wooded area, while in the built area it was at a lower level and more variable. This would suggest that the demand for inhibition, the expense of cognitively applying the brakes in the built environment, can indeed be a drain on attentional resources among the children.

In a separate study from the University of Illinois group, children with diagnosed attention deficit disorder (ADD) completed a series of challenging puzzles to increase their directed attention fatigue before setting out on a guided walk for 20 minutes. In keeping with the methods in these recent studies, one group subsequently walked through a lush park within an urban setting, another in a downtown area, and a third in an area clustered with houses. The researchers ensured that the three environments had similar amounts of graffiti and garbage, were all relatively flat, and had low levels of ambient noise and pedestrian traffic. The walks were also conducted under similar weather conditions. After the 20-minute walk in one of the three environments, the children were driven back to a quiet indoor setting for a series of objective measures of attention and executive functioning. The results were clearly in favor of the natural setting as a cognitive enhancer—the children who had walked in the park knocked it out of the park: the improvement in cognitive function matched that reported for the two top-selling ADHD medications.

## Anger and Impulsivity

The fallout from mental fatigue isn't merely a personal matter relevant only to the fatigued individual. Overtaxing the brain sets the stage for increased anger and impulsivity, and this in turn sets in motion a cascade of negativity in all manner of interpersonal interactions. The frustration and strain of mental fatigue primes an individual to react to anything and everything perceived as negative—and when an individual is mentally fatigued, every environmental stimulus seems magnified in its negativity. The person who walks around the office or schoolyard quick to anger will not win friends and positively influence people: negativity breeds negativity. The tentacles of attention deficit are far-reaching and can ultimately compromise family, work, scholastic, and basically all social relationships. Given the importance of social connectivity in human health and well-being, the implications are enormous. Even the mere perception of social isolation is associated with diminished cognitive functioning.

In modern society, one of the most prevalent and dangerous ways in which one can take out negative energy is on the road. Approximately one-third of North Americans admit they have experienced road rage—shouting, gesturing at the occupants of other vehicles, or driving in an aggressive manner. These incidents commonly occur with high traffic density and are more common after clocking up many miles on a given day. Without doubt, the incidents are fueled by stress, frustration, and fatigue.

Nature might be a component of a road rage vaccine of sorts. A 2003 study showed that the amount of vegetation along a highway can help mitigate driver frustration. Here again, the volunteers were cognitively fatigued with mental challenges up front before proceeding on a simulated drive where the modified variable was roadside vegetation. The participants had a much higher frustration threshold after "driving" on roadways with more vegetation in sight. After the simulated drive, the researchers had the participants work at a complex mental problem. Interestingly, those who "drove" on the high-vegetation parkways worked at a difficult post-drive mental challenge for a much longer period than those who had "driven" in the built areas. This is the heart of mental fatigue: frustration builds up and the individual gives up on the task at hand; he or she is no longer motivated to pursue the goal. This finding was essentially a cognitive validation of reduced frustration among these participants. Less fatigue on the road translates into more cognitive sharpness and tolerance of others.

Impulsivity is the tendency to take swift action without foresight and planning, and is often caused by a deficit in the inhibitory pathways of the brain. It's like a scene from a 1980s action movie: a car races down a winding mountainside road while the driver stamps frantically on the brake pedal, but nothing happens—the brake line has been cut. When we are mentally fatigued, the brakes, or inhibitory centers of the brain, are exhausted and don't keep impulsivity in check. When we are impulsive we make risky choices and seek short-term rewards without considering long-term goals and rewards. Impulsivity can influence food choices and retail purchases (and subsequent credit card balances); at a more extreme end of the continuum, it is associated with addiction, suicide, and serious violence. Being prone to impulsive action impedes the ability to make healthy lifestyle modifications despite one's best intentions.

Nature, it seems, can repair the brake line and provide the fluid refill to help keep anger and impulsivity in check. Research has shown that viewing

- scenes with significant amounts of vegetation (regardless of rural or urban setting) is associated with lower reported anger levels,
- higher amounts of nature from apartment-building windows is linked to greater scores of self-control (lower impulsivity), and
- greater vegetation through windows had a big impact on girls (average age of 9): they were more willing to put off short-term rewards for longer-term benefit, performed better on tasks of concentration, and had higher scores of impulse inhibition.

### Dr. Eva's File

Alex, a junior in college, was an "anxious mess," according to his mom. Finding that Alex's ADHD medication only made him worse, she felt at a loss to help him and so had come asking for my help. She complained that Alex was unable to concentrate and would likely fail his classes, as he spent the majority of his days playing video games or sleeping. Alex for his part said that he was "addicted" to video games because it was easier to concentrate on the screen than deal with the overwhelming anxiety he experienced when thinking about his school-work. In his first two years of college he managed to get mostly Bs. Now, in his junior year, he could barely pass. What changed between his sophomore and junior years, I wanted to know, since, according to Alex, the classes were not necessarily more difficult.

At the end of his sophomore year, two things happened. His long-time girlfriend broke up with him and he received an Xbox for his birth-day. Initially, he found solace and escape in the on-screen world and battle. He stopped going out with friends and even going outdoors. He couldn't remember the last time he enjoyed himself being around other people, and felt social anxiety at the mere thought of it.

So I asked Alex to recall a time of happiness being out in nature, not necessarily with people—perhaps doing a sport. Without thinking, he answered, "When I'm skiing or hiking in the mountains."

"So, how about it?" I asked. "How about I give you a prescription to go take a hike for 15 minutes a day to start?"

Alex laughed but then grew serious and agreed to the plan.

He started with 15 minutes and over the next few months found himself gradually spending more time hiking and skiing and less time playing with the Xbox. As his anxiety and feelings of being over-whelmed started to disappear, he reported that he could concentrate better on his schoolwork. He still enjoyed playing with the Xbox, but he realized that it was actually a great activity to enjoy with friends, one that helped him overcome his social anxiety.

## Indoor Plants and Cognition

In the 1980s, researchers began to accumulate data that indicated that positive affect (i.e., how one feels at a given moment) can have a ben-eficial influence on cognitive organization. Specifically, they found that brief periods of positive affect (induced by simple means such as a small gift, a five-minute comedy film, a word-association game with positive words, or a juice-and-cookies refreshment) enhanced an individual's ability to visualize connections or interrelatedness between objects, boosting that person's creativity. A good mood allows one to see the big picture and to respond favorably when faced with new challenges and information, whereas distress, anxiety, and anger decrease one's ability to cognitively turn on a dime, so to speak.

Researchers conducted the first formal investigations on plants and office performance in Japan. Two separate studies showed that the presence of potted plants in the vicinity of a computer workstation reduced eye strain and operator fatigue. After this initial work, North American researchers reported that the mere presence of potted plants improved productivity and reaction time among adults tested on a computer task involving visual concentration, mental processing, and manual dexterity. Immediately after the computer test, the participants were queried on their perceived levels of attention; those in the room with a small selection of plants reported significantly higher levels of attention than their study counterparts. In a similar study, researchers at the University of Illinois manipulated a test room by having no vegetation, a few potted plants (10 total), or a lush setting containing 22 plants (close to 20 percent of the office space). The participants completed a series of productivity tasks in one of the three settings, after which they completed subjective surveys. Although the participants in the high-vegetation room reported the highest degrees of comfort and perceived attractiveness of the environment, they also had the lowest productivity scores, worse than those in the room with no plants, indicating that an office space should not be transformed into a virtual tropical forest—the participants seemed to be too comfortable for work! In the moderate-vegetation room, there was a balance between mood and performance.

A more recent investigation highlights the value of just a few plants in the office setting. Here, the researchers compared a no-vegetation room to one manipulated by adding only four plants (two small flowering plants on a window ledge, a one-foot-tall green plant on the desk, and a four-foot-tall floor plant). The participants were asked to perform memory recall and complex proofreading exercises. Those in the plant room showed improved performance between baseline and an evaluation 10 minutes later. Furthermore, Japanese researchers manipulated a small office and reported that the presence of a four-foot-tall corn plant improved mood and performance scores among women on a task designed to evaluate creativity.

Interior plants have been shown to improve subjective learning, behavior, and health in academic settings, particularly in classrooms without an adequate number of windows. And as we go to press with this book, researchers at the University of Technology in Sydney, Australia, have confirmed that indoor plants placed in a classroom can make a meaningful difference to academic scores among younger students. Specifically, the researchers placed three plants in half of the middle-school classrooms in three Brisbane school districts. Over 350 students were involved in the study, all of whom completed standardized academic tests prior to the plant installation and again six weeks after the plants were placed in select rooms. Significant improvements in mathematics, spelling, and science were reported in the students who had plants in their classrooms. The improvements ranged from 10 to 14 percent, reflecting a meaningful difference—any positive change of 10 percent or more is generally regarded by education professionals as a significant indicator of student progress.

Obviously, a few potted plants are not going to put someone into the express lane to becoming a card-carrying Mensa member; we understand their limitations. Still, we simply cannot ignore the potential cognitive edge that plants might provide in our increasingly competitive school and work environments. Based on the research to date, if nature, even in its reduced form of potted greenery in the workplace, can stimulate a small degree of happiness and reduce stress, then indeed we have a factor worthy of investigation and investment beyond mere aesthetics.

## The Future of Nature and Cognition

Although nature appears to acutely benefit cognition, the long-term consequences of your brain on nature may be even more important. Greenspace is clearly a means of improving mental outlook and reducing the stress burden in the body, and as such it will have long-term benefits in keeping the brain as sharp as possible through the aging process. Depression and low-grade stress are a corrosive force, a sort of rust that attacks brain cells, accelerating the normal pace of aging in the brain. Nature, on the other hand, has the potential to encourage the growth and continued reshaping of the brain cells throughout life, improving the brain's so-called plasticity.

This is the future of the cognition-nature research: to provide proof that time spent in nature can influence the production of brain chemicals responsible for maintaining cognitive health through the aging process. At least one study has already shown that walking in a forest environment (versus same time spent walking in an urban environment) is associated with a significant elevation in the neurosteroid dehydroepiandrosterone (DHEA). This was an important finding because DHEA declines with aging, and its administration has been shown to improve cognitive performance in adults. DHEA encourages the subsequent production of other chemicals—or nerve growth factor production—and the preservation of cognitive sharpness through the aging process. Healthy older adults with the highest levels of brain nerve growth factors are resilient against cognitive decline. Among older adults, DHEA levels have been reported to be lower in association with the modern Western lifestyle. Since the stress hormone cortisol interferes with DHEA production, a link to lower DHEA and higher stress and anxiety through the aging process should not be surprising.

The stress of city life is not a friend of cognitive health. Gerontologist Dr. Martha Sanchez-Rodriguez reported in a 2006 issue of *Life Sciences* that urban residence is a risk factor for cognitive impairment through the aging process—as much as five times greater than rural residence. Specifically, when her team compared groups of healthy, well-nourished urbanites and rural controls 60 to 80 years old, they found that the rural residents scored better on mental tests used to evaluate cognitive decline and clinically relevant cognitive impairment through the aging process. They also found that the urban residents had higher blood markers of oxidative stress versus the rural residents, and that oxidative stress itself was highly linked to cognitive impairment. Oxidative stress, as previously discussed, is a corrosive force in the brain, one operating in tandem with psychological stress. It remains an open question as to what degree urban greenspace, gardening, and forests can help to buffer against age-related cognitive decline. Based on the early hints, there is every reason to suspect that nature, probably more effectively than a hand-held "brain game," can temper the degree of cognitive decline in urban settings.

# 4

## Something in the Air: Specific Elements of Nature on the Brain

*The fragrance with which one is feasted in the woods is, like music, derived from a thousand untraceable sources...the whole air vibrates with myriad voices blended that we cannot analyze. So also we breathe the fragrant violets, the rosiny pine and spicy fir, the rich, invigorating aroma of plushy bogs in which a thousand herbs are soaked...*

—John Muir

Although it's clear, as the discussions in the previous chapters illustrate, that nature can provide benefit to psychological outlook and internal stress physiology, scientists are often inherently drawn to investigate at the microlevel. Simply viewing various nature scenes in an MRI scanner can capture the visual sense; yet, true nature immersion is an experience that can stimulate all of our senses. Scientists have not been content to simply accept the environmental link between visual nature and the workings of the brain; over the years they have dug deeper to determine whether specific elements of nature influence emotions and physiology. They have determined that beyond mere aesthetics and visual perceptions of beauty, nature can indeed stimulate the senses by way of specific variables, including plant-derived aromatic chemicals, natural light and colors, various sounds, and negatively charged molecules called negative ions.

As more and more people move toward an urban life, a greater understanding of how we can leverage some of nature's more potent elements, particularly as a way to buffer the stress of contemporary life, is a worthy scientific pursuit. It's not always so simple to escape the urban artificiality for a jaunt to the woods to get yourself that much-needed forest bath. A small dose of a specific element of nature may provide immediate calm and focus when stress and tension are rising. In putting together the scientific puzzle of our innate relationship to nature, the results of these more reductionistic investigations are underscoring the many ways in which we are intimately connected to countless minute aspects of the natural world.

## The Aromas of Nature

In recent years, scientists have made stunning discoveries about the delivery of various drugs, including hormones, vaccines, and compounds with small peptide units, through the nasal route. They now recognize that the intranasal pathway is a potential route of entrance to the brain for a much wider variety of substances than once thought. Incredibly, nasally administered substances, including plant-derived vapors, are capable of entering the brain and then exiting into body-wide blood circulation.

Greenspace provides untold amounts of olfactory-provoking chemicals that appear to act synergistically, balancing mental outlook and facilitating effortless attention to the environment in which one is immersed. You can usually smell flowering plants, but even though a single tree of a single species can release several dozen aromatic chemicals, your sense of smell commonly fails to detect them. But just because they escape overt detection by your sense of smell does not mean they are without consequence to health. Collectively, these individual aromatic components are called phytoncide. Some of the individual components stimulate, while others sedate, so engaging in a forest bath (shinrin-yoku) exposes you to the entire constellation of aromatic chemicals, which can uplift and relax the brain. Experimental studies have shown that phytoncide produced from trees can lower the production of stress hormones, reduce anxiety, and increase pain threshold, while inhaling aromatic plant chemicals increases the antioxidant defense system in the human body. They have also shown an association between higher amounts of phytoncide in the air and improved immune function. Specifically, higher levels of airborne phytoncide cause increased production of anticancer proteins in the blood as well as higher levels of the frontline immune defenders called natural killer cells (NK cells). When we are exposed to viruses (e.g., influenza, common cold) and other infective agents, NK cells step up to protect us. Indeed, adults who have higher NK activity have lower frequency of colds. The work of physician Qing Li of Nippon Medical School in Tokyo has been groundbreaking. He has shown that on days when aromatic phytoncides (derived from Japanese Hinoki cypress trees) are aerosolized into hotel rooms, study participants have lower levels of stress hormones and increased NK activity versus control days. Business travelers and those traveling for an important interview or presentation can easily appreciate the significance of the findings. Furthermore, Li's team has shown that a weekend shinrin-yoku trip (walking one and a half miles twice per day) improves NK activity not only for a day or two; rather, compared with those walking in a pleasurable urban weekend control trip, the NK activity remained higher for an additional month. Even a day trip for forest bathing (in a suburban forest north of Tokyo) improved NK activity, with significant differences over baseline lasting for a week. Trees and plants secrete aromatic chemicals that impact our cognition, mental state, and even our immunity in ways we are only just beginning to understand. Isolating the individual aromas that aid with human wellness allows us to have more focused treatments with real-world significance to those beyond study participants. Here again, science is verifying something our ancient ancestors seemed to know well.

## Airborne Aromatic Chemicals

For at least 4,000 years, aromatic plant extracts—wood- and flower-derived resins, gums, oils—have been prized and used for a wide variety of medicinal, religious, dietary, and ceremonial purposes. Ancient Greek physicians recognized that the aromas of certain plants tended to be stimulating, whereas the inhalation of other groups of plant-derived oils was reported to have a sedating effect. Ancients used airborne aromatic plant chemicals for ceremonial purposes to solidify the emotional connection felt by participants; the scents aroused the participants' senses and enhanced their mental acuity and relaxation so they felt more fully present in the moment.

Although once lumped in with the stuff of crystal balls and black capes adorned with half moons and stars, aromatherapy and its application in human cognition and mental health disorders is now receiving increased interest from the scientific community. Large reviews of existing aromatherapy data show that in randomized controlled studies on anxiety and depression, subjects reported a meaningful reduction in symptoms, and the aromatherapy was safe and well tolerated. Experimental studies have shown that plant oil vapor can enhance the production of the brain's own calming chemical gamma-aminobutyric acid (GABA), while also boosting mood-regulating serotonin function.

Some of the more intriguing aromatherapy studies highlight the polarizing ways in which aromatic plant chemicals can influence the brain—some, such as rosemary and lemon oil, stimulate; others, such as lavender and rose oil, are more sedating. While walking through the forest can be both uplifting and relaxing thanks to the natural combination of plant aromas, aromatherapy offers an opportunity to fine-tune the advantages offered by selecting individual plant aromas. For example, a 2002 study conducted in the United Kingdom showed that workers toiling in cubicles scented with rosemary had significantly better memory recall than their colleagues who worked in unscented cubicles or cubicles scented with lavender. In fact, workers in the lavender-scented cubicles demonstrated diminished working memory and performed poorly on attention-based tasks compared with those working in unscented cubicles. So workers hoping to graduate from cubicle to corner office might do well to avoid lavender until after work, when they can use it to unwind.

Researchers at the Wheeling Jesuit University have conducted numerous studies in the realm of natural aromatic chemicals. They have reported that peppermint improves both physical and mental performance. When subjects inhaled very small amounts of peppermint, their typing speed and accuracy improved, as did their alphabetization performance. They also performed better on attention and memory-testing tasks and reported less fatigue than subjects who inhaled cinnamon or jasmine aromas or no scents at all. These same researchers also discovered that peppermint and cinnamon aromatherapy might just bring one back from the brink of road rage. In their experiment, the researchers found that prolonged driving led to increases in anger, fatigue, and perceptions of physical demand, as well as decreased vital energy. Peppermint and cinnamon decreased driver frustration and increased alertness; peppermint alone lowered the levels of anxiety related to extended driving. Interestingly, the aroma of fast food and pastries, both frequent companions on the road, aggravated drivers' frustration and increased their willingness to speed.

In a study published in the *International Journal of Psychophysiology* in 2005, researchers at Coventry University, United Kingdom, found that jasmine may promote sleep quality and increase alertness the following day. During their three-night investigation, researchers exposed students to one of three conditions: jasmine scent, lavender scent, or no scent at all. Specifically, they infused the students' rooms with the scent of lavender or jasmine at such low levels that many of the students were completely unaware of any scent at all. Not only did the jasmine sleepers toss and turn less frequently, they woke up feeling less anxiety. The jasmine sleepers also performed better on cognitive testing the next day. (Lavender was good too, but it couldn't match jasmine.) A recent study involving sophisticated brain imaging (fMRI) has reported that even without specific instructions to rate pleasantness and intensity, minute levels of jasmine aroma can enhance activity in the areas governing attention.

Research shows it takes only miniscule amounts of these aromatic chemicals to provide health benefits. Indeed, when it comes to aromatherapy, less appears to be more. For example, Japanese researchers reported that *low* levels of jasmine aroma can dampen down an overactive sympathetic nervous system—the stress branch of the nervous system. But those who told the researchers up front that they did not like jasmine had an *increase* in activity of that branch of the nervous system when exposed to high levels of jasmine scent.

## Plants as Vacuum Cleaners

Just as natural aromatic chemicals surround us in greenspace, human-made synthetic chemicals surround us in more urban areas, creating unnaturally polluted environments. And just as surely as miniscule levels of inhaled natural plant chemicals influence the brain, so too can synthetic chemicals. However, synthetic airborne chemicals and overt unpleasant odors typically have a negative influence on cognitive and emotional health. Exposure to indoor and outdoor airborne pollutants in residential and occupational settings has been linked to anxiety, depression, autism, aggression, irritability, pain, fatigue, frustration, short- and long-term cognitive decline, decreased altruism, and an overall downturn in individual helping behavior. Ambient air pollutants can set in motion a cascade of low-grade inflammation and have recently been linked to type 2 diabetes, cardiovascular disease, and obesity. Here, we are just referring to the obvious sources of outdoor air pollution from heavy industrial factories and traffic. Additional chemicals emitted from building material and the contents of buildings, including furniture, electronics, carpet, paint, cleaning supplies, vinyl flooring, faux wood, plastics, and air "fresheners," also impact us negatively. Recent studies show that ambient air within indoor urban settings contains volatile chemicals, most notably benzene and formaldehyde, at levels that are beyond guidelines set by expert panels.

The computers in our homes and offices have been shown to contribute significantly to total indoor levels of toluene, 2-ethylhexanol, formaldehyde, styrene, and other potentially nasty chemicals. In a 2004 study, researchers at the Technical University of Denmark unpacked six new computers and operated them for 500 hours. Three weeks later they placed the computers behind a room divider. Otherwise healthy adults were randomly asked to perform cognitive tasks in identical workstations while unaware of either the presence or absence of the half dozen computers behind the divider. In the meantime, the researchers measured the air quality of the room while keeping air temperature, lighting, humidity, noise level, and air flow constant. The results of cognitive testing showed diminished performance and increased errors in those rotated through the workstations close to the hidden computers. The amount of volatile chemicals in the ambient air was significantly higher in the room with relatively new computers. The results confirmed a similar study where a decline in indoor air quality, due to a hidden chunk of polyamide-fiber carpet, diminished office performance in a series of randomized cognitive tests.

Here again, plants may come to the rescue, acting as a sort of vacuum cleaner for the air. While most people understand that plants and trees provide the oxygen we need, the role of nature as a cleanser tends to be underappreciated. In the late 1960s and early 1970s, researchers published several articles showing that certain trees and other plants (petunias, for example) were not only resilient against smog, they were able to significantly lower the levels of airborne environmental pollutants. Scientists such as Paul E. Waggoner made note of the great potential of plants, and trees in particular, as a way to purify polluted air in metropolitan settings. In the ensuing decades he has been proven right—plants are well capable of handling environmental chemicals, metabolizing and transporting them to the soil where subsequent bacterial action can render them less harmful.

In the 1980s, a few years after environmental scientists established that various trees and plants could act as pollution solutions, and after they discovered some 107 nasty volatile chemicals within the air of their Skylab, NASA scientists stepped into the plant-air-purifying arena. The NASA group used the air-purifying properties of plants as a way to allow astronauts to remain healthy while working and living in enclosed spaces constructed of synthetic materials. Before the installation of the indoor potted plants, high levels of airborne volatile chemicals were emitted from the synthetic materials in the enclosed testing facilities, and sickness was frequently reported. Installing the plants quickly removed the volatile organic chemicals from the air and diminished the typical respiratory and eye irritation.

Since the first NASA reports, numerous studies published in scientific journals have shown that various plants can bring about a massive reduction in the amount of airborne volatile chemicals within offices and other enclosed spaces. Indeed, the potted plants involved in the investigations reduced indoor pollutants by 75 percent or more. Considering that urban dwellers spend 90 percent of their time indoors, these investigations have tremendous relevance to our health and well-being. However, this does not mean that we should be abusing plants and trees by using their absorptive strengths as an excuse to dump more synthetic chemicals into the air. Just because plants can soak up pollution for us—some 700,000-plus metric tons per year in the United States—it doesn't mean they should.

### Depression—A Gray and Odorless World

When patients with depression are asked to pick out their favorite color, like healthy adults, they opt for a mid to light shade of blue. However, when looking at 38 color options, those with depression are far more likely to associate their current mood state with three shades of gray. Compared with healthy adults, twice as many individuals with depression equate their mood with a color. Those with depression aspire to see "the blues" while they suffer with grays.

A study published in 2010 in *Biological Psychiatry* explains why that might be—patients with depression have difficulty discerning the contrast between black and white: things literally look more gray, and the greater the severity of depression, the worse the difficulty with contrast. Add to this, research showing that patients with depression have smaller olfactory bulbs (which are responsible for smell) and a diminished capacity to detect minor scents in the air, and it becomes clear that those with depression perceive the world differently. Separate studies have linked impairments in the processing of smell and other sensory information to anxiety and ADHD. These findings underscore the need for additional nature therapy to treat depression. In fact, those with depression may have the greatest need for nature-based immersion—natural light, colors, and aromatic scents.

## Light—Natural Deprivation and Artificial Gluttony

Timing is everything, the saying goes, and when it comes to the human relationship with the nonvisual aspects of light, this is especially true. There is much more to light than its essentiality in vision. Light hits the retina and sets off a cascade of biophysical events unrelated to vision. The interaction between environmental light and the light-sensitive cells in the retina is far-reaching and can ultimately influence sleep, alertness, mood, and cognitive performance. For some 2 million years, humans have been groomed on a steady supply of natural light from the sun, and the transition from morning light to evening darkness was the chief environmental signal for the brain's 24-hour cycle of arousal and sleep.

Natural light in the visible spectrum enhances cognitive performance during the day, and the withdrawal of light, in the transition from evening to darkness of night, brings about a decline in mental performance and an increased desire to sleep. The advent of electricity and the invention of the lightbulb gave us the option to extend the day and light up the skies. Burning the midnight oil became the rule for societies, rather than the exception. Today, more than half of the world's population lives under a night sky far brighter than nature allows for even with a full moon. While a full 20 percent of the urban workforce works at night, a much larger percentage are at home and technically off the clock, yet they too are illuminating their retinas as they "work" the screen. Modern computer monitors and plasma TVs can be very bright; in fact, flat-screen TVs can be 20-plus times brighter than a 60-watt bulb.

In contrast to our floodlit nights, we spend our daytime hours in environments that are often devoid of adequate natural light. Certainly, our use of artificial illumination can help to get us through our days, but we still don't get enough of the cognitively enhancing and mood-supporting visible light provided by nature. The typical indoor office cubicle provides a worker with artificial light some 100 times lower than midday winter sunlight. For workers confined to desks during the shorter days of winter, particularly at northern latitudes, this lack of natural light can contribute to melancholy. Our timing with light, it turns out, is quite the opposite of what it should be; we miss out on our daily fix of natural light, particularly during the winter months, and a few hours later we light up our eyes at a time when nature's darkness is telling us to wind down.

The connection between darkness and sleep, mediated via the hormone melatonin, is hard-wired within us. The production of melatonin is inhibited by light and enhanced by darkness. Production increases in the mid to late evening when the light begins to dim. Secretion and levels in the blood peak between 2 a.m. and 4 a.m.—some 20-fold higher than daytime levels. Studies have shown that it doesn't take much late evening or nighttime light to adversely affect melatonin production—flat-screen TVs and computer monitors boast about brightness, and their 400 to 1,000 lux can cause a sharp fall in normal melatonin production. Just 30 minutes of exposure to 400 lux illumination or two hours of 300 lux can significantly reduce nocturnal melatonin levels. You might be thinking that the 60-watt bulb used for reading is just as bad, or what about the oil lamp, the candle, and the hearth fire used by our ancestors? Not so much. These all produce illumination in the range of 20 to 60 lux and have very little effect on melatonin production.

There are massive consequences to the artificially brightened night sky. Recent experimental research shows that even low levels of light during the night can reduce brain plasticity and interfere with normal adult brain cell structures. And the health consequences, compounded by our interrupting the normal production of melatonin, include associations with insomnia, immune deficits, cancers (most notably breast cancer), obesity, daytime fatigue, attention deficit disorder, irritable bowel syndrome, fibromyalgia, and depression. Scientists are vigorously investigating the use of oral melatonin as a therapeutic agent in many of these conditions.

## Light as Therapy

> *Why is it called "after dark" when it*
> *really is "after light"?*
> —George Carlin

Physicians have advocated purposeful exposure to natural light as a therapeutic intervention in mental health disorders for centuries. Two thousand years ago, Roman medical experts not only advocated therapeutic garden walks for those with mental illness, they also recommended that those with melancholy and chronic digestive problems live in spaces filled with light. In the early 20th century, clinical reports of improvement in mental health symptoms via exposure to the ultraviolet, infrared, and visible (light) portions of the electromagnetic spectrum began to accumulate. Hospital in-patient treatment plans widely discussed the use of southern-exposure windows to maximize natural light in patient rooms. However, despite the popular use of solariums, southern-facing windows, and machine-generated electromagnetic light therapy, there was little in the way of clear biological explanation for the beneficial outcomes.

It wasn't until the 1980s that researchers began to make consistent connections between low melatonin levels and depression. The early research focused on the use of bright-light therapy in those most sensitive to the shorter winter days—people with seasonal affective disorder (SAD). These early light therapy studies have since accumulated into volumes of international research clearly in favor of its value, and in 2002, Australian researchers confirmed sunlight plays a direct role in the production of the mood-regulating brain chemical serotonin, the very brain chemical drug companies have been attempting to elevate via Prozac and all of its chemical cousins. They found that the rate of serotonin production was directly related to the daily duration of ambient sunlight.

Now that researchers have determined that light therapy works to reduce SAD, they've turned their attention to additional considerations, including the appropriate dose and wavelength of light. Solar radiation arrives to earth as visible light, and the relatively slight variations in wavelength dictate the color that we actually see. The latest research suggests that the blue portion of the visible light spectrum, the very portion that shows the greatest relative decline in winter (compared with the longer wavelengths green and red), is most influential in mood states. The artificial light cast by traditional bulbs provides very little of the blue spectrum. Clinical intervention studies using blue-enriched white light or blue light (e.g., a goLITE BLU table-top and travel-portable light therapy box) suggest that mood symptoms can be improved without the hour or two required at 2,500 lux or the intense use of 10,000 lux with traditional units. For example, the goLITE BLU can provide results at 1,000 lux in as little as 15 minutes of exposure during the winter months. The gains produced by light therapy are not marginal: depression ratings have decreased by as much as 82 percent.

Given the broad therapeutic potential of oral melatonin and the mood benefits of bathing our brain cells in just a hint more serotonin, light therapy researchers have looked beyond SAD, examining other mental and cognitive health issues. Recent investigations have reported that light therapy is valuable in relieving other forms of depression, eating disorders, and anxiety. While SAD is relatively rare, occurring in 1 to 5 percent of the populations living at northern latitudes, a seasonal change in mood during the transition to winter is not uncommon. As many as one in two adults report a downgrade in mood and mental outlook when the dark winter days encroach and the clocks fall back. With hemispherical consistency, people type the word "depression" into the Google search box at far higher rates during the winter months. Looking at five years' worth of global Google data over 54 geographic locations, researchers found that regardless of language, typing in the word "depression" and clicking on the Search button was dependent on season and latitude. During their summer, North Americans took a relative break from searching sites related to depression, while at precisely the same time, Australians were again back to the high level of depression queries. This underscores the notion that light deficiency might be its own syndrome, one that influences a greater portion of the population than that captured by the SAD diagnosis. It also suggests that light therapy, if provided at the right time and not via a flat-screen TV at 10 p.m., could benefit a significant group of people who sit just below the diagnostic criteria of SAD.

Light therapy (1,000 lux) in the morning can improve cognitive functioning, alertness, subjective happiness, low-grade anxiety, and subsequent sleep in otherwise healthy adults. More specifically, recent studies have again identified blue light as enhancing certain aspects of cognitive functioning over green, red, and violet portions of the spectrum. Studies using fMRI have shown that the blue portion of the light spectrum can specifically fire up areas of the brain that involve attention and memory. In a 2008 UK study conducted in the winter, blue-enriched white light was installed on one floor, while similar fluorescent tubes not enriched with blue were added on a different floor. Assessment four weeks later among 100 office employees revealed that the blue-enriched light improved mood, performance, alertness, irritability, and evening fatigue. The subjects on the blue-light-enriched floor also reported sleeping better at night, suggesting that they were keeping melatonin well suppressed during the day and taking advantage of daytime performance benefits without compromising sleep (such is not always the case with energy drinks and coffee). Unlike standard fluorescent tubes, blue-enriched fluorescent tubes provide the wavelength we need during the winter months, and thankfully they are now becoming more widely available (Phillips's Master TL5 ActiViva is one type).

The beneficial light used in the study was not merely blue; it was the full visible light spectrum *enriched* with blue, therefore it also included colors in the red and green ranges. Light completely devoid of red, orange, yellow, and green can influence brain functioning. Sophisticated brain imaging studies have shown that exposure to the green portion of visible light alone can deactivate certain areas of the brain. In 1903, *Medical Age* reported that select Russian prisoners were kept in rooms devoid of the red, orange, yellow, and green portions of the natural visible light spectrum. It was a form of torture without physical pain. After prolonged periods, the subjects were depressed and cognitively exhausted.

---

### Blue Light and Suicide Prevention

In 1877, G.L. Ponza, director of a mental asylum in Alessandria, Italy, made international headlines when he reported preliminary work with colored lights and their influence on his patients. *Canada Lancet* stated that "the results attained by the use of blue and red lights were remarkable, the former quieting and soothing the patients into a calm condition, and the red exciting to violence." In particular, blue light was said to produce its most profound effects in those with high levels of mental agitation.

Over a century and a quarter later, in 2009, executives from the East Japan Railway installed $200,000 worth of blue LED lights at select Tokyo train stations in an effort to curb suicides. Although no specific scientific research indicates that blue light can reduce suicides, contemporary studies do suggest that blue light can have immediate effects in brain cell communication, including those involving the emotion fear and fear-related behavior. Research shows that those who make violent suicide attempts have impaired decision-making processes in the brain. Blue light temporarily improves cognition and enhances responses to emotional stimuli, and brain imaging studies indicate that it can be an acute jolt to the system. For a despondent individual standing on the edge of the platform, the functional brain changes induced by blue light might be to the brain what defibrillation paddles are to the heart during cardiac arrest.

## Why We Need Windows

Despite the wonderful advances in artificial light therapy, we cannot overlook the simple adjustment that requires no electricity: leveraging the value of simple windows. Indeed, not only do windows provide visual access to the outside world but they are the portal for therapeutic delivery of light from the sun. In the mid-1800s, it became clear that windows in the classroom, particularly south-facing windows, could play a role in the acceleration of academic progress. Writing in an 1869 issue of the *Journal of Education for Ontario*, school superintendent Newton Bateman stated that "neglect of the common principles of optics in providing and arranging light in school-houses is a common evil." Even with the mass introduction of artificial light, natural light from windows was held in higher esteem for the educational environment, and up until the 1950s, schools relied on natural lighting to a large degree. Yet, in the late 1960s and 1970s, the tide turned, based on a short-sighted and erroneous view that windows were energy-wasteful. Skylights were covered up, buildings were retro-fitted with fluorescent bulbs, and designs became radically different. Windowless was the new trend.

Although glass might be back in vogue, the low natural light in many of these old school buildings remains, and the damaging effects persist. If we want our children to thrive in school, they need a view to nature and an access point for the sun to shine in. In recent years, windows in classrooms have been shown to enhance concentration, particularly during the winter months when children have less exposure to outdoor natural light. An investigation involving 21,000 students in three geographic locations (Seattle, Washington; Fort Collins, Colorado; Orange County, California) reported that students in classrooms with the largest window areas progressed as much as 15 percent faster in math and 23 percent faster in reading than students in classrooms with few windows.

The office is another environment in which windows are of critical importance. Workers in underground settings without windows have been found to be more anxious, hostile, and depressed than their colleagues on the windowed floors. Happiness is defined as having a preponderance of positive thoughts, and those working in windowless offices are more likely to experience negative thoughts in the course of the workday. As long as glare and temperature can be controlled, windows are highly prized by office employees; promotion to the corner office usually comes with financial compensation, more responsibility, and lots more natural light. Research indicates that employees sitting closer to windows are more content than their colleagues who sit closer to the core of a floor. Enhancing the level of daylight within interior workplace environments has been linked to improved productivity in a wide variety of industries. Of course, windows facilitate a certain view, be it of bricks or greenspace. People working in office settings would rather have a smaller window with a nice view than a large window with a not-so-nice view, yet any window is preferable to no windows in a workplace. While a view to nature can obviously enhance the mood and cognitive performance of employees, simply allowing sunshine into the interior space has been associated with increased job satisfaction, well-being, and intent to stay with an organization. Importantly, these latter findings were above and beyond illumination per se. In other words, it had nothing to do with brightness; it was letting some sunshine in that really mattered.

In health-care settings, windows provide a bridge to the outside world. In her nursing manuals, Florence Nightingale made specific references to the benefits of natural light and fresh air afforded by windows. She stated that there should be a maximum of two beds per window, and that patients should be elevated as much as possible so that they could see outside. She writes, "*Window*-blinds can always moderate the *light* of a *light* ward; but the gloom of a dark ward is irremediable." Further, patients should "see out of a *window* from their beds, to see sky and sun-*light*." Studies from 1996 and 2001 have shown that high levels of natural sunlight can expedite recovery and reduce the length of hospital stays in patients with either major depression or bipolar disorder. In patients treated after a heart attack, those who were assigned rooms with high amounts of natural light were more likely to recover faster, and amazingly, there was a 7 percent difference in mortality rates in favor of the rooms with high levels of natural light. Furthermore, in another chance finding, postoperative patients who had undergone spinal surgery reported less stress and lower pain levels, and used 22 percent less pain medication than post-op patients placed in rooms on the other side of the hospital—the side that happened to have 46 percent less natural light.

The benefits of windows are not exclusive to in-patient rooms: two studies have reported that even small windows in the intensive care unit are associated with less frequent delusions, hallucinations, and depersonalization post-recovery. Patients and hospital employees alike rank windows high on the list of desirable building features; of course, the view from those windows is also an important part of the equation. We have come a long way since Florence Nightingale's advice, and now bedside windows are often mandated by government regulations for hospital stays beyond one day. Indeed, large windows and rooms with a view to nature are now routine bragging points in hospital marketing literature.

## Negative Ions

Negative ions are charged molecules that we cannot feel, see, smell, or taste. The level of these molecules that we inhale is dependent on the environment that surrounds us. Negative ions are found in abundance in forests and near bodies of moving water. Negative ions in the air, molecules carrying an extra negative charge due to nature's splitting action, are yet another unseen and underappreciated aspect of outdoor natural settings. Researchers recently linked the regional abundance of negative air ions to improved human health and longevity. But negatively charged air ions, which are prevalent in natural settings, can become quickly depleted within polluted external environments, as well as in enclosed and air-conditioned rooms. Negative ions are also lowered by electronic devices found in homes and offices, such as computer screens, photocopy machines, and televisions. For example, the air in copy centers contains almost five times more positive ions than outdoor air on the same day.

According to research published in a 2004 edition of *Indoor Air,* negative air ions have been shown to promote our antioxidant defense system, lower blood lactate levels, and improve aerobic metabolism by enhancing blood flow. In an intriguing study published in the *Canadian Journal of Anesthesia* in 2004, a negative ion–generating machine was placed in a hospital setting where minor skin surgeries were conducted under local anesthesia. Unbeknownst to the patients, the machine was switched on or off during alternating weeks; humidity, temperature, and other background factors were controlled. Other than the local anesthesia, none of the 95 patients received medication. Psychological tests showed that those who had been exposed to the negative ions had less tension and a more rapid reduction in stress associated with the procedure.

Beyond the minor surgery study, various investigations have shown benefits of negative ions in reducing stress, depression, and anxiety, and improving cognitive performance. Research published in 2005 in the *International Journal of Biometeorology* shows that patients prone to panic attacks are much less likely to experience panic after a rainfall, when negative ion count is high. Researchers have been able to provoke anxiety, suspicion, and mania in environments with an absence of negative ions. Interestingly, the seasonality of ADHD, generalized anxiety disorder, depression, and panic disorder—all worse in the winter—may be to some degree influenced by the lower levels of negative ions found in the air during winter months. The föhn of Switzerland, Austria, and southern Germany and the chinook of Alberta have long been connected to irritability, headaches, and low-grade depression. These dry winds are distinct in their relative absence of negative ions. With the exception of post-rainfall, negative air ions are at their highest during clear, calm days with not too much or too little humidity. Since negative ions peak in the morning around sunrise and again during the late evening, walking in natural environments during these times could potentially be even more beneficial to your brain.

---

### Jet Lag—Beyond Time Zones

Do you ever feel out of sorts after a flight? Most often this is, with good reason, blamed on jet lag; however, the aircraft cabin air itself may be a brain-changer. The humidity is very low inside aircraft cabins, the negative ion content is at low ebb, and ozone levels can be very high, sometimes double the World Health Organization's eight-hour guidelines. In a four-hour simulated flight, ozone levels comparable to what have been found on commercial flights (60 to 80 parts per billion) were associated with mental tension and more significant feelings of claustrophobia versus a low (less than 2 parts per million) ozone flight.

---

## Water

> *The underlying attraction of the movement of water and sand is biological. If we look more deeply we can see it as the basis of an abstract idea linking ourselves with the limitless mechanics of the universe.*
> —Sir Geoffrey Jellicoe

Much like green vegetation, water can play a direct role in our mood and cognitive restoration. Fresh water has always been required for our survival, and we have not been shy at taking advantage of the nutritional riches found in salt water environments. Various anthropologists have posited that the expansion of brain size and evolution of humans was driven by marine-derived fatty acids found in fish and shellfish.

Our attraction to water is evident. Both children and adults consistently rank water environments among their favorite places, and vacations and leisure activities often take place in aquatic environments. A water view can drive up real estate prices beyond the norm. When researchers at the United Kingdom's Plymouth University asked 40 adults to rate over 100 pictures of green natural and built urban environments, the respondents gave higher ratings for positive mood and preference to any photographic images containing water, regardless of environment (although greenspace, as expected, trumped the urban built environment). Interestingly, there was a consistent attraction to water up to a certain point—scenes containing between 33 and 66 percent water were, as Goldilocks would say, just right. Too much or too little water detracted from preference scores.

The healing powers of water have been promoted since Roman and Greek physicians used specific protocols to treat various ailments. In the late 1800s and early part of the 20th century, hydrotherapy became part of standard care for mental health disorders. In the 1920s and 1930s, hospitals featured specific hydrotherapy departments specializing in mental health care. Physicians used immersion in warm water or alternating hot and cold water, exposure to warm water vapor, warm and cold wraps (wet packs), and steady stream showers with varying degrees of success in treating depression, anxiety, fatigue, and mental exhaustion. In any case, with the advent of psychiatric drugs and talk therapy, hydrotherapy as a mental health modality was largely washed up by the mid-20th century.

Thankfully, a small group of contemporary researchers have tried to shed light on some of the physiological mechanisms whereby hydrotherapy might influence mental health and emotion. Immersion in warm water, it turns out, is akin to meditation in its influence on the central nervous system. Objective investigations have shown that warm-water bathing improves the balance between the branches of the nervous system governing stress and ultimately promotes activity of the "rest and digest" (parasympathetic) branch. The researchers have shown that the act of floating in warm water, so-called flotation therapy, reduces levels of the stress hormone cortisol, muscular tension, and cardiac rate, and improves emotional state. Objective testing has also shown that patients with anxiety disorders who were immersed in warm water experienced reduced muscular tension and improved symptoms of anxiety within about 15 minutes.

A series of recent Japanese studies indicated that warm-water bathing, bathing with added micro-bubbles of air, and the direct application of a mild stream of water over the legs and back while bathing all reduce physiological markers of stress and mental fatigue while improving mental outlook and cognitive performance. Separate Japanese investigators found that even warm footbaths could enhance sleep by improving stress-dampening branch (parasympathetic) activity. And combining airborne plant aromatic chemicals with water can enhance the effects. For example, lavender in a warm footbath maintains parasympathetic activity for a longer period than just a footbath alone.

## The Sounds of Nature

*In the attitude of silence the soul finds the path in*
*a clearer light, and what is elusive and deceptive*
*resolves itself into crystal clearness. Our life is a long*
*and arduous quest after Truth.*
—Mahatma Gandhi

Finding a remote spot in a natural setting can be an acoustical paradise. You might hear birds singing, creek water splashing on rocks, a twig breaking under hoof or paw of an animal, wind whistling through leaves or pine needles as trees sway…you get the idea. These sounds of nature are 180 degrees away from the sound waves emanating from a leaf blower, a jet aircraft, a helicopter, construction equipment, vehicle horns, and all the other artificial waves causing a modern-day acoustic smog in our urban and suburban environments. Noise is a plague, and although most of us know that high volume on our headphones or hanging out near a jackhammer can damage our hearing, the low-grade stress induced by noise-producing machines continues to be underappreciated. Environmental noise promotes the production of stress hormones, places a burden on the cardiovascular system, compromises cognitive and academic performance, depresses the immune system defense, contributes to insomnia, and enhances the likelihood of depressive thoughts and anxiety. Ultimately, environmental noise catches up with us: we now know that prolonged exposure to environmental noise can decrease longevity itself.

The imprint of 2 million years of nature contact on the contemporary human brain has been evidenced again as recent studies confirm that we detect and process nature-based sounds in different ways than we do modern sounds. One might presume that human-made alarm sounds—rapid-succession high-pitch sounds that provoke urgency—would lead to immediate attention in the contemporary brain. Yet, a study published in 2010 in the *Journal of the Acoustical Society of America* showed that natural sounds—from a lion, leopard, or jaguar, for example—produced faster reaction times than classical warning tones. On the other hand, natural sounds such as flowing water and birds chirping can mask the perception of road traffic and construction noises. The introduction of natural sounds turns down the annoyance factor of environmental noises. In office settings, nature sounds—wind, rain, stream water, ocean waves, birds—can mask steady machine noises, and employees prefer them over a setting without nature sounds. Hopefully, researchers will have a closer look to determine if this masking technique using natural sounds can put a dent in the harmful physiological effects of environmental noise.

Some studies have looked specifically at nature sounds as a means of lowering stress. In a 2010 study from Stockholm University, adult volunteers experienced brief mental stressors interspersed between sounds of road traffic noise or nature sounds (water and birds). A more rapid normalization of physiological markers occurred when the background noise involved nature sounds. In hospital settings, exposure to natural sound has been associated with better sleep in patients post cardiac surgery, lowered stress hormones during surgery, and pain reduction during bronchoscopy. The Japanese research team from Chiba University, shinrin-yoku experts Drs. Yoshifumi Miyazaki and Juyoung Lee, have shown that the sounds of a creek induce changes to brain blood flow indicative of a state of relaxation. The blood flow changes are in direct opposition to what is usually observed with mental stress and exhausting cognitive challenge. In addition, researchers have determined that listening to recorded bird sounds early in the morning can lift mood and decrease fatigue. In those with sleep difficulties, it also may help reset normal production of the sleep hormone melatonin.

National parks, forests, and wilderness areas remain our last bastion of noise refuge, and respondents en route to such areas often state that escaping from noise is a primary motivation for their visit. As interesting as the potential of natural sounds to mask urban noise might be, the converse is perhaps even more interesting: when machine noise comes to nature, the distress is amplified. Put simply, the annoyance factor when technological sound waves encroach into natural settings is very high. Machine-derived noise can quickly undo many of the positive attributes of nature discussed thus far. Nothing can dampen the restorative and mood-lifting influence of natural settings quite like the noise of a machine. Aircraft, traffic, chainsaws, landscaping equipment, motorboats, or motorcycles— all detract from positive perceptions of natural settings. In contrast, the sounds of nature, birds chirping, and water flowing enhance the positive mental outlook associated with nature scenes. Therefore, we cannot assume that all the previously discussed benefits of greenspace are due to green per se—the contextual acoustics might just make or break the mental benefit. Cities are expanding and acoustic energy is increasing—some cities have doubled their acoustic energy levels since 1990. Given that trees, particularly evergreens, provide superb insulation against noise, we should consider expansion of greenbelts and urban forests as one of the many steps we must take to limit our metropolitan noise problem.

---

### Instant Mood Changer—Light, Sound, and a Chaser of Some Negative Ions

How rapidly can some of the natural elements we have discussed—bright light, sounds, and negative ions—influence mental outlook? Do these nature components, collectively known as environmental therapeutics, change mood in a rapid fashion? Research published in *Psychological Medicine* in 2006 suggests that using a light box (10,000 lux), a birdsong melody mix on CD, or a negative ion–generating machine can indeed facilitate mood change within 15 to 30 minutes, compared with a placebo, which was ineffective. These active components of nature reduced depressive thoughts and total mood disturbance among healthy college students at a meaningful level—a 41 percent average improvement from baseline mood, as well as reductions in anger. Obviously, such mood changes will only help to facilitate cognitive functioning and creativity. Hopefully, researchers will examine the effect of bright light, sound, and negative ions together in an effort to determine a synergistic effect.

For more on the use of negative ion generators and different light boxes, as well as self-assessment tools, visit the Center for Environmental Therapeutics website at www.cet.org.

---

# 5

# Green Exercise Is Like Exercise Squared

*It is not the walking merely, it is keeping
yourself in tune for a walk . . . when the exercise of
your limbs affords you pleasure, and the play of your
senses upon the various objects and shows of nature
quickens and stimulates your spirit, your relation to
the world and yourself is what it should be—simple
and direct and wholesome.*

—John Burroughs in *Pepacton*, 1881

Records suggest that organized exercise has been used as a formal means of health promotion for some 4,500 years. Ancient Chinese texts and the recommendations of the best-known Greek and Roman physicians (Galen, Hippocrates, and Celsus) made clear references to the importance of physical activity for optimal mental and physical health. In the mid-1800s, the first scientific suggestions that a physically active lifestyle was a disease repellant were published, observing that tailors, confined to an indoor seated occupation, had a significantly shorter lifespan than outdoor laborers working on farms. Although many factors other than physical activity could have accounted for the difference—air quality, dietary habits, light exposure, vitamin D, and so on—the study suggested that sitting around might be deadly. Similar studies followed in the early part of the 20th century, including comparisons between bus drivers who sat all day long and bus conductors who would walk throughout the day, indoor administrative postal clerks and mail carriers who walked neighborhoods, and white-collar office workers and physically active manual laborers. All showed that occupational sitting is a disease risk factor, particularly for cardiovascular disease.

In the 1920s and 1930s, physicians wrote formal prescriptions for exercise in general and, more specifically, outdoor exercise, as a means of improving physical and mental health. A so-called physical culture grew into its own entity, and gymnasiums began to expand in metropolitan centers. But there was still a general sense that physical activity in fresh air (parks, for example) could trump indoor exercise. Experts such as George L. Meylan, a Columbia University physician and president of the American Physical Education Association, stated that the benefits of exercise alone could be amplified when conducted in natural environments.

As with many other branches of lifestyle medicine, exercise became a victim of the pharmaceutical boom of the 1950s and 1960s. Incredibly, despite the historical enthusiasm for exercise and the large population studies indicating its benefits, even in the 1960s experts debated whether exercise was a health promoter. At best, exercise was a secondary or tertiary talking point, far removed from frontline drugs. Who needed exercise when scientists were on the verge of discovering a workout in a pill? In the age of science, evidence was lacking, and the famous Wolfenden Report, published in 1960 in the United Kingdom, examining sports and exercise, concluded that "we have not found any unequivocal connection between taking exercise and being healthy." In 1963, exercise proponents, including physiologist professor C. Mervyn Davies of the London School of Hygiene and Tropical Medicine, lamented the lack of science with which to direct policy.

Thankfully, in the span of 40 years, all that has changed. Volumes of international research now provide irrefutable evidence that regular physical activity is effective in the prevention of a variety of chronic diseases, including cardiovascular disease, obesity, diabetes, certain cancers, depression, and osteoporosis. Exercise is now a formally recognized medicinal agent. Scientists can now look to other pressing issues, such as ways to tear down the barriers to physical activity and to promote adherence to exercise, while also examining in further detail the ways in which exercise works to promote health. Furthermore, scientists are investigating whether outdoor exercise in natural settings—so-called green exercise—provides an added edge over the city sidewalk or treadmill. With the advances of science, researchers in various medical branches are making remarkable discoveries about the specific effects of exercise on the brain. They are also showing that Columbia University's Dr. Meylan was right: green exercise is like exercise squared.

## The Cognitive Benefits of Exercise

Evolutionary biologists have taught us that the human body is designed for movement: for more than 2 million years, our unique shape allowed us to beat out the competition for food. Before there was a drive-thru window and delivery within 30 minutes or it's free, humans were rewarded for movement via sustenance. The mental reward for movement is alive and well today, if only we can get past the obstacle of motivation to fitness. Exercise is one of our most important brain tonics, and its benefits are available to everyone, from early childhood through the golden years. Exercise improves cognitive functioning— manifest, for example, in academic grades, creativity, perceptual skills, memory recall—and acts as a mood-regulating stress buffer. Among large groups of healthy 5-year-olds, those who are the most aerobically fit have the highest scores of attention, and those who have the best balance also have the most efficient working memories. Can you imagine the market value of any medicinal agent that could foster attention and working memory? Both of these attributes are solid predictors of academic achievement, which in turn can predict to some degree how life will unfold. This life-unfolding business is not mere speculation; a recent study reported remarkable findings on data derived from over 1.2 million males involved in compulsory screening for Swedish military service. The researchers found that aerobic fitness in early adulthood (in this case, 18 years old) predicted higher educational achievement and socioeconomic status later in life compared to young adults not aerobically fit.

Recent findings on brain fitness take on enormous implications given the widespread sedentary nature of our screen culture. In the largest study of its kind, published in 2007 in *Medicine and Sport Science,* when researchers analyzed data from 27 nations since 1958, they found the aerobic fitness numbers looked great through the 1970s. But we've seen a steady drop since, and in particular there has been a marked decline in aerobic physical fitness among children aged 6 to 19 during the last two decades. Recall from Chapter 2 that IQ gains in developed nations may not only be leveling off, they may even be in decline as fitness declines and the screen moves in.

---

### Exergaming—Good, but Not as Good

Some contemporary video games promote active participation in the form of dance and sports games. Obviously, this is a major step up from playing a war game while the waist expands on the couch. Exergames can get the blood pumping and burn up calories; some even qualify as a moderate-intensity workout. But when it comes to the exercise benefit of cognitive restoration—recharging the brain—good old running appears to have an edge. In a head-to-head comparison of treadmill running with exergaming at similar duration and intensity, the running group had enhanced cognitive performance in the area of attention control. Specifically, the ability to block out unimportant and distracting information was subsequently enhanced by traditional running. The inference is clear: nature-based exercise may provide a much-needed cognitive advantage in an overly distracting world.

The good news is that fitness is a modifiable risk factor: we can do something about it. Improving aerobic fitness can improve cognitive functioning in both the young and old, and not just in speed of processing information but in critical aspects of executive function that really matter in academic achievement and social functioning. Physical activity, even relatively short bouts, can improve our ability to filter out irrelevant information, increase working memory, and help us make associations. Exercise doesn't just enhance cognitive response time; it increases the accuracy of the response. In the modern world, any intervention that improves one's ability to eliminate distractions and stay on task with accuracy is invaluable. In a social setting, an inability to filter irrelevant information in the face of multiple tasks puts an individual on the fast track to saying or doing something without inhibition. This can happen regardless of age; however, the inability to inhibit and filter is a hallmark of the older brain, at least one not fortified by the protective factors of physical activity. As the brain ages, the inhibitory pathways are easily overwhelmed, and this seems to be why older adults have a propensity to say what they really think. Their lack of inhibition causes them to overlook social consequences. Aerobic fitness is associated with focused attention to the relevant matters at hand, while at the same time bolstering the inhibition centers more efficiently.

Scientific support for exercise, particularly the simple act of walking, as a cognitive protectant is strong. Large studies have shown that walking may be one of the most effective ways to keep the brain cognitively fit. Dr. Jennifer Weuve and colleagues from Harvard showed that among 18,000 older adult women, walking was associated with significantly better cognitive function and the prevention of cognitive decline. In separate work, Dr. Robert Abbott of the University of Virginia found a similar effect in over 2,200 older males. Men who walked the least had an almost twofold increased risk of dementia compared with those who walked more than two miles per day. The benefits of walking are not restricted to the brains of older adults— consider that in children and teens, walking for 20 minutes increases subsequent stress resiliency and cognitive focus. Walking to school has been linked to higher academic performance in junior and high school–age girls, a research connection that became very strong among girls with a walking commute longer than 15 minutes.

## Exercise and Mental Health

International research clearly indicates that physical activity is an antidepressant and antianxiety agent, showing that both acute and long-term exercise can improve mental outlook, alleviate mild-to-moderate depression just as surely as medications and counseling, and decrease sensitivity to anxiety and panic attacks. Suffice it to say that exercise as an intervention has been well documented to positively influence mental state.

When low-grade daily hassles accelerate into major depressive disorder, physical activity declines. This loss of physical activity can prolong recovery and, of course, it sets the stage for physical conditions that are two- to threefold higher in those with depression: cardiovascular disease, type 2 diabetes, and osteoarthritis. It really becomes a vicious cycle because the reverse is also true: lack of physical activity predicts depression. When researchers followed over 10,000 healthy young adults (without mental health disorders or medication use at baseline, that is, at the outset of the study) for six years, they found that those who spent the most time in front of screens such as television and the Internet were over 30 percent more likely to subsequently develop a mental health disorder compared with those who avoided such activities. When it came to actually engaging in physical exercise, those who were among the most physically active decreased their odds of a mental health disorder by 28 percent.

Even moderate levels of physical activity (exercise activities, such as a brisk walk or gardening, during which one can still maintain a normal conversation) are associated with positive psychological well-being. Exercise provides a buffer against stress, and those who report regular exercise are more resilient to illness during times of elevated stress. Aerobic exercise has been shown to decrease the subsequent reporting of health-corrosive daily hassles. Researchers at the University of California, San Francisco (UCSF) demonstrated the dramatic potential of exercise as a stress buffer and cell protectant in 2010. They looked at cellular components known as telomeres—small caps that insulate and protect genetic material, much like the plastic tips on the end of a shoelace. The telomere length is correlated to the potential life span of the cell, and shortening is associated with an increased risk of damage and cellular death. Unsurprisingly, short telomere length has been linked to numerous chronic diseases and early mortality. Chronic stress, and a higher degree of perceived stress, has been associated with shorter telomere length, whereas exercise has been linked to longer telomere length. The UCSF researchers wanted to determine if there was an interaction between stress, exercise, and telomere length. Incredibly, even after controlling for a host of lifestyle and socioeconomic factors, they found that exercise could completely erase the connection between stress and telomere length. Among healthy nonexercising adults, perceived stress was highly linked with short telomeres, whereas 40 minutes of vigorous activity eliminated the association between perceived stress and telomere length. In a stress-filled modern world, the implications are, of course, enormous. According to American Psychological Association annual surveys, stress perceptions are at an all time high; an intervention that can block its corrosive force is certainly worthy of the doctor's prescription pad.

## How Does Exercise Promote Brain Health?

Scientists began to examine the physiological pathways of exercise and its brain benefits by focusing on the ability of exercise to promote the production of "feel good" and pain-reducing brain chemicals such as serotonin and opiates. Recently, it has become clear that exercise does indeed influence a wide range of mood-regulating neurotransmitters. In fact, the latest studies show that exercise alters serotonin production in ways that are quite similar to antidepressant drugs. Moreover, exercise has been shown to increase the production of the nerve growth factors that facilitate normal brain cell structure and functioning.

These nerve growth factors, including a key brain-protecting chemical called brain-derived neurotrophic factor (BDNF), have direct antidepressant properties. In addition, exercise encourages the production of chemicals that control the integrity and growth of blood vessels. In short, exercise supports blood flow to the brain, which in turn encourages even further production of the chemicals that take care of our brain cells.

Paradoxically, although exercise initially turns up the dial on both inflammation and oxidative stress, when it becomes incorporated into a regular part of lifestyle habits, it has both antioxidant and anti-inflammatory effects. In untrained individuals, an acute bout of exercise can initially amp up the production of inflammatory chemicals, and free radical production becomes rampant. This is part of the "no pain, no gain" mantra while initiating an exercise protocol. However, an adaptation process takes place. With a little time and experience, moderate exercise improves the body's overall antioxidant defense system, and fitness becomes a resiliency factor against chronic low-grade inflammation.

Numerous studies have shown that classic blood markers of low-grade chronic inflammation are low in those who are physically fit, and clinical exercise interventions can put a dent in the burden of body-wide inflammation. Even a two-hour walk through a forest can reduce chemicals linked to depression, cardiovascular disease, and inflammation. The levels of a key inflammatory chemical linked to chronic disease, C-reactive protein, are three and a half times higher in sedentary versus physically fit adults. Some of these inflammatory chemicals can compromise a healthy mental outlook. When healthy, physically fit individuals give up their exercise routines, they begin to experience fatigue, irritability, tension, and depressive symptoms.

## The Benefits Are in Your Mind

Undoubtedly, there is a placebo response built in to the reported benefits of exercise. Serotonin and other mood-regulating brain chemicals can influence attitude, but the release of these chemicals can be triggered by exercise or by simply inducing a change in mental outlook. For example, provoking happiness and positive thoughts can elevate brain serotonin levels, whereas provoking sadness can decrease them. The expectations, beliefs, and perceptions about exercise can ultimately promote its benefits. In a Harvard study published in 2007 in *Psychological Science,* researchers informed one group of employees that the physical activity they were doing was vigorous enough to meet governmental guidelines for activity. The subjects in the other arm of the study were given no such verbal information, and the physical activity was identical between the groups at both the outset and the conclusion of the study. What was remarkable was that, after four weeks, the informed group perceived themselves to be more fit and did indeed have lowered blood pressure, weight, waist-to-hip ratio, and body mass index versus those in the noninformed control group. For many scientists, these sorts of findings diminish the luster of exercise, somehow taking away its "scientific" credibility. However, we see things differently: the mind-body connection becomes a potential reinforcer for an intervention that protects mental and physical health.

Does it really matter if exercise is 50 percent perception and 50 percent physiology? Not really, according to the research. Perception becomes an individual's reality. Consider that large population studies have shown that perceived health reported by older adults is at least as good, and often better, as a predictor of longevity than are objective measures of health status. If expectations and beliefs are encouraging people to get out the door and move, then so be it. In a world where sedentary screen time is the rule and not the exception, we encourage more expectations, more beliefs, and positive perceptions concerning exercise.

## Adherence—Promoting the Brain Benefits of Exercise

Physical activity can, if practiced consistently, lift the mood, lower anxiety, and provide a coat of armor against daily hassles and the corrosive forces of stress. There are three words in the preceding sentence that act as a qualifier, an asterisk, the fine print: "if practiced consistently." And therein lies the problem—for the most part, it's not. And incredibly, the very latest studies have made it clear that we have been *overestimating*, if you can believe it, the extent of physical activity among North Americans of all ages. In two separate Canadian nation-wide studies, one involving adults and the other children and teens, participants wore a device so that researchers could accurately and objectively measure daily physical activity. These were not small stud-ies: there were close to 3,000 adults (age 20 to 79) and 1,600 children and teens (age 6 to 19) of various backgrounds recruited from 15 sites across Canadian provinces—a group representing a well-balanced slice of North America. The results were not pretty, with only 15 percent of adults meeting the guidelines set by the World Health Organization (WHO) of 150 minutes of physical activity per week. Only 7 percent of the children and teens met the WHO guidelines set for this age group: 60 minutes of moderate to vigorous activity per day. What can we do to change this, and can green exercise help?

When it comes to compliance with even short-term prescription medications, human beings average only about 70 percent adher-ence. Sadly, the reality of noncompliance with prescribed physical activity programs is even worse, with as many as two-thirds throwing in the towel. Surely there is a way to increase the odds of compliance, to alter the mind-set related to exercise from "must do" to "look forward to." There is always a segment of the population who just love to exercise—they look forward to going to the gym, jumping on the treadmill, and perhaps taking a specific exercise class. This relatively small minority of highly motivated individuals are driven in large part by the identity factor. Exercise becomes part of their very being—just as surely as they might be a chef, a lawyer, or an engineer, so too are they identified as a runner, a cyclist, a skier, or a gym rat. They are also motivated by pride, ego, and, more importantly, health-promoting outcomes. Surprisingly, the exercise-induced "feeling states," as psychologists call them—the positive and happy thoughts, the refreshed mental attitude—are not the deciding factor in exercise engagement and adherence for the highly motivated.

On the other hand, for the folks who are not inclined to exercise, those with lower self-motivation scores, the exercise-induced feeling states become *the* central story when it comes to sticking with aerobic exercise. Positive thoughts, tranquility, mental revitalization, and other measures of mood changes induced by exercise are much more important—10-fold higher—to the larger segment of the population, the individuals who otherwise find it difficult to put down the remote and get off the couch. For the majority of us, these mood or affective changes can become a dynamic motivator, acting ultimately as a bridge between good intentions and actual behavioral change. Still, a quandary remains. When sedentary adults have time to reflect upon turning intentions into behavioral change, they tend to think of the negative. Indeed, the preponderance of negativity may not even require reflection. Those who are sedentary are more inclined to have immediate, rapid-fire negative mental associations with words linked to exercise—researchers say "jog," they think fatigue; researchers say "athletic," they think exhausted; and so on. When people are already in a time-pressured, fatigued state, these automatic associations can dictate behavior and offer a magnetic pull toward the couch.

Even though exercise is a well-proven method to improve general fatigue, we must first overcome the negative mind-set. We must also overcome some of the inevitable negative thoughts associated with the physical difficulty of initial bouts of exercise—just as surely as positive mental thoughts can drive the sedentary adult to stick with an exercise routine, a preponderance of negative thoughts (achy, fatigued, tired, worn-out) can rapidly extinguish all good exercise intentions. Researchers call this a nocebo response—negative outcomes result from negative expectations, which is basically the opposite of the placebo response. The key is to magnify the positive emotions, particularly during the early "no pain, no gain" period when absolute sedentary activity becomes moderate to vigorous. This is where green exercise can work its magic, amplifying positive thoughts, tranquility, and cognitive refreshment at the very time when individuals need it most, and thus diminishing the pain and enhancing the gain.

# Green Exercise Trumps the Treadmill

*The gymnasium, athletic track, and the swimming
pool are ameliorators to our synthetic modern living
but they are not the same as the rocks, rivers and
trees. The Greeks knew that the sea was for the
swimmer and the earth for the feet of the runner.*

—Professor Peter J. Arnold, Chelsea College of Physical Education, 1970

The outdoors in general, and greenspace in particular, is a great facilitator of physical activity, with research showing that neighborhood access to greenspace is a significant predictor of moderate to vigorous physical activity. For example, electronic monitoring demonstrates that children who go outside to play will have a two-and-a half-fold increase in physical activity, which is an obvious deterrent to obesity.

Researchers comparing indoor and outdoor exercise have found one clear reason why people with access to the great outdoors are more inclined to exercise: it makes them feel better. In 1980, famed psychologist James Pennebaker and colleague Jean Lightner designed an experiment wherein they set up a level 1,800-meter (1.12 mile) running trail through woods and another 1,800-meter level trail in an open, nonwooded area. Adult subjects, all of whom were novice runners, were asked to self-select a pace and jog the courses (all subjects jogged on both courses in alternating fashion over a 10-day period) without knowing the intent of the study until its conclusion. The results showed that jogging through the woods resulted in faster completion times, more satisfaction, more enjoyment, and less frustration than the open laps. While jogging in the woods, the research subjects got outside their internally focused thoughts and instead directed their thoughts to the outside world of the wooded environment. This resulted in decreasing perceptions of fatigue and physical symptoms that otherwise interfere with exercise.

In 1990, Japanese scientist Yoshifumi Miyazaki of Chiba University and colleague Yutaka Motohashi provided a more detailed look at the mood changes and differences in objective stress physiology between indoor and outdoor exercise. They set up a walking experiment in Japan's forest jewel of Yakushima, a World Heritage site rich in a wide variety of evergreens and with the greatest plant biodiversity in Japan. The subjects walked for 40 minutes in a forest setting and on a separate occasion, on a treadmill in a laboratory. Based on the subjective paper and pencil reporting, compared with the treadmill, the forest exercise elevated mood and vigor while lowering fatigue, tension, and anger. The researchers also correlated the subjective reports of the forest walk benefits with reductions in blood pressure and the cortisol levels compared with the treadmill. Miyazaki has been examining shinrin-yoku exercise with even more vigor over the last five years, and along with colleagues Juyoung Lee and Qing Li, they have been bringing portable medical equipment into field settings. Together they have shown in numerous studies in dozens of Japanese forests that walking in forests (a total of four hours per day split into segments versus similar time spent urban walking) lowers blood pressure and stress hormone levels, and enhances the activity of the "rest and digest" (parasympathetic) branch of the nervous system. The latter observation comes from the use of a portable device measuring heart rate variability (HRV), a simple yet effective tool for examining the activity of the nervous system under stress.

Other studies confirm the findings of Pennebaker and Miyazaki that outdoor exercise boosts mood and reduces stress:

- Research involving one-hour walks showed that in middle-age adults, a rural walk improved mental outlook and was more cognitively restorative versus an urban walk of the same duration. The study, published in a 2011 issue of *Health and Place*, showed that after the walks, those who entered the study with the highest levels of emotional stress had the highest gains in cognition and mood. The results suggest that those dealing with high levels of stress have the most to gain from the green exercise experience.

- In a study published in *Medicine and Science in Sports and Exercise* in 2011, research subjects were asked to select a pace and walk on an indoor treadmill or an outdoor track. While walking outdoors, subjects chose a faster pace, had more positive thoughts, and perceived less overall exertion versus walking on the treadmill. This translates into a happier, less-tired individual who is ultimately burning more calories.

A study of experienced runners published in 1995 in *Psychophysiology* found that running outdoors versus on the treadmill at an equivalent duration is associated with less fatigue, diminished anxious thoughts, less hostility, more positive mental thoughts, and an overall feeling of invigoration.

In addition to encouraging activity through these positive mental effects, outdoor exercise appears to improve one's athletic performance. In the early 1980s, Soviet sports scientists examined records related to athletic performance within closed gymnasiums and open-air settings—noting that in the majority of head-to-head matchups, outdoor performance was trumping indoor. They suggested that the factors we covered in the previous chapter, most notably airborne plant chemicals (phytoncides), were at play. More recently, in a 2011 study, researchers at Texas State University evaluated the competitive performance results of 128 track-and-field athletes during a spring competition season. The subjects were drawn from Texas universities, and the four major event locations where competitions were to take place were rated on a greenness scale. Results showed that surrounding greenness was indeed a predictor of best performance.

Even the quality of exercise improves when you head into nature. Researchers are discovering that a forest offers a better training environment than the gym. Running in open air provides a varying degree of resistance to the runner and, even with little wind on a calm day, the small increase in energy expenditure required to fight the wind can add up over time. Running through a forest—versus on a treadmill or pavement—also requires extra effort because of its natural undergrowth and varying gradients. Walking through a forest trail or cross-country running in natural environments provides an ever-changing surface—soft soil, hard soil, sand, embedded rocks, tree roots, decaying vegetation, fallen branches, and so on. Emerging research suggests that both the physical and brain benefits of exercise may be enhanced by making contact with uneven surfaces. Nonuniform surfaces encourage the activation of many muscles of the legs and ankles, muscles that may be underutilized in a perfectly flat, human-made environment. Research shows that standing on a shifting, slightly uneven surface reduces fatigue, prevents the pooling of blood in the lower limbs, decreases the stress placed on the cardiovascular system, and keeps more blood up in the brain.

### The Joy of Climbing Trees

To take from boyhood the legitimate pleasures and adventures of tree climbing would unduly restrict the confines of that memory cherished domain, and lessen life's joys, both there and thereafter.

—1919 Maine Supreme Court ruling against Lincoln County Power Company

Just about all kids love to climb, and it is easy to see their joyful feeling of conquering the limbs of a pine tree. This childhood climbing desire may indeed be written into the human DNA. Before we had ladders, ropes, cranes, and mechanized cherry pickers, we still had a hungry desire for eggs, fruit, honey, and other nourishment found in high places. In our 2-million-year communion with nature, a post-meal feeling of satiation was often dependent on tree-climbing skills. For children, the joy and happiness typically outweighs the fear of the climb, and this serves to keep the drive alive.

Around the time that the Maine Supreme Court was ruling on the joy of tree climbing, its popularity among adults was on the rise, with tree climbing being promoted as a form of exercise for both mind and body. Today, there is a new wave of supervised tree-climbing programs, complete with modern safety techniques and devices to ensure that the joy factor outweighs the fear factor—and these programs are growing in popularity.

Since it may be difficult for youthful urban dwellers to legally take it upon themselves to start scaling local trees, an emerging intervention called tree-climbing therapy is starting to take root. The experience is not only the act of climbing trees per se; it also incorporates mindful contemplation of making nature contact. Tree-climbing therapy (also called tree-assisted therapy) has been the subject of recent scientific investigations in Japan. Results show that tree climbing in the therapeutic sense reduces tension and anxiety while also improving mental clarity and feelings of vitality. Interestingly, when compared with climbing a human-made structure with artificial branches, the climbing of a real living tree was associated with higher scores of vitality and energy, as well as lower scores of tension and cognitive confusion.

In addition, the findings show that participation in tree-climbing programs fosters an increased concern for the environment and motivate subjects to be involved in efforts toward its conservation.

For more, visit the Tree Climbers International website at www.treeclimbing.com.

## Putting Research into Motion—Practical Solutions

### Dr. Eva's File

Peg hated to exercise. At 52 years of age, she proudly stated that she never had to exercise, since she had been able to maintain her weight by eating healthy foods—up until menopause, that is. Over the past four years, she complained, the weight had started to piled up, especially at her midriff. She knew the only way to keep the weight off was through exercise, but no matter what she tried, she couldn't stick to a regimen. She simply hated it. She had even hired a personal trainer a few times but quickly lost her enthusiasm.

Knowing Peg lived near a beautiful reservoir, I suggested she try mindful walking for at least 30 minutes a day, appreciating the beauty and bounty of what she observed in nature. This way, her focus would be taken away from the exercise and what she did not enjoy, and directed toward appreciation of what she could enjoy.

Along with her drive to lose the extra weight, Peg was able to stick to this exercise regimen. In fact, she even found a walking buddy with whom to enjoy nature's beauty.

The notion that exercise is a medicinal agent for mind and body is scientifically sound. We contend that green exercise can magnify the general benefits of exercise, offering a natural Zoloft effect, and this perspective is gaining research-based support. However, there comes a time when research needs to be put into practice. Unless we actually get out there, it will remain a stack of data. Based on the existing research, we have compiled the following advice regarding dose and delivery of medicinal green exercise:

1. **Self-selection.** The same protocol used by doctors for initial prescriptions of antidepressant medications applies to exercise: "Start low, go slow." When individuals self-select the pace (the walking speed, for example), they are more likely to enjoy and stick with an exercise routine than they would if the routine were prescribed, with high expectations. Pushing the exercise envelope a little bit is okay. However, it becomes a problem if the intensity of the exercise is itself a source of psychological stress. When researchers invoke psychological stress during an exercise routine in otherwise healthy adults, they observe a marked elevation in stress hormones, oxidative stress, and inflammatory chemicals. Viewing exercise as a forceful and distasteful endeavor defeats its purpose. Interestingly, many laboratory animals enjoy taking advantage of running wheels, jumping on and off them at will. And when they do so, the physiological benefits such as elevations in the brain-protective

chemical BDNF become apparent. Not so when these same animals are "told" when and how to exercise. When voluntary exercise becomes involuntary, the brain benefits appear to diminish—even in rodents.

2. **Standard duration and intensity.** Perform 30 minutes of moderate-intensity outdoor physical activity at least five days per week, or a total of 75 minutes per week of vigorous activity. Moderate physical activities are those that get the heart and breathing rates up a bit but don't interfere with conversation. If you walk a forest path with a friend, you can still have a conversation if walking at a decent pace. If you are running on the forest path, your heart rate and breathing are elevated even further, and it becomes difficult to have a conversation—you have now put yourself into vigorous activity mode.

3. **Setting goals.** You needn't become a marathon runner or a triathlete. A good walk or a light jog in greenspace may be just what the doctor ordered for your brain. Make an effort to increase the pace of a walk within your own comfort levels. Experts in exercise for brain benefits suggest setting a realistic goal of 8,000 steps per day and ultimately moving up to the widely proclaimed 10,000 steps. Keep in mind that 10,000 steps is five miles, which can be a lofty goal for those with depression or anxiety—they may be averaging only 2,000 to 3,000 steps per day in conjunction with a sedentary lifestyle. At this point, any level of physical involvement is a good beginning. The short-term goal is incremental yet manageable progress in a graded fashion. Mood elevation and anxiety reduction can be found with as little as 20 minutes of exercise, and this will assist in pushing you toward longer-term health goals. One of the longer-term goals might be to reach the clinical "antidepressant dose" of exercise—that is, a level of improvement that is in line with the expectations of standard medication and cognitive behavioral therapy. The final goal in mental health dosing is ultimately a bit higher than average

recommendations: walking for 45 minutes five days per week, or jogging 38 minutes five days per week. Again, this is a goal that can be gently achieved in graded fashion over time. In those with depression, too much too soon typically serves to pour water on the already diminished sparks of motivation.

4. **Matching.** To strengthen the likelihood that you'll stick with exercise, choose activities that reflect your preferences. Don't run if you prefer to walk. Swim if it enhances the joy of exercise and minimizes the post-exertion fatigue. Also choose an environment you enjoy. It can be green (lots of vegetation) or waterside (by a creek, river, lake, or ocean), but keep in mind that a combination of green and water has emerged as the most valuable exercise environment in terms of elevating mood and self-esteem.

5. **Accounting.** Draw up a scheduled plan with short- and long-term goals, and then keep a record of what you do, including frequency, duration, and any pertinent notes on your mind-set associated with a particular exercise and its setting.

6. **Assistance.** To increase the chances of success, including adherence to and the enjoyment of your exercise regimen, check in with a coach, therapist, or exercise professional. Have him or her help you stick to a schedule and problem solve to overcome barriers to exercise consistency. When physicians prescribe tailored advice in writing, with details about local areas for exercise opportunities and ways in which to advance physical activity, adherence is maximized. Some mental health professionals, or ecotherapists as they are sometimes called, now conduct counseling sessions while walking within greenspace. We discuss this in some detail in Chapter 9.

7. **Make time.** Undoubtedly, longer working hours are commonplace. The screen is a time thief, work spills into the home, and parents, especially working women, feel tremendous pressure to devote quality time to family members. Where to fit in

exercise? Think of green exercise as an investment in yourself. In order to come even close to fulfilling modern-day expectations, you must make your mental and physical health a priority. Green exercise improves mood and vitality, busts fatigue, and decreases tension, stress, and anxiety, so while it serves you, it also benefits all those you come into contact with—including children, spouse, in-laws, and coworkers. Put simply, green exercise is worth making time for, and, in truth, there is always time. It becomes a matter of priorities. Research shows that total working hours per se are not the deciding factor in whether adults engage in physical activity.

8. **Alone or together?** Green exercise can be conducted with friends and family or alone. There is some research indicating that in healthy adults, outdoor exercise is more relaxing and reduces overall stress when conducted alone. Sometimes immersion in nature and contemplation while exercising solo is a cleansing activity; being alone is what is needed to charge your mental batteries. But there are times when exercise with a friend or a group can amplify the benefits by encouraging social connectivity. For those with mental health disorders, group walking in nature has been described as a healing balm for the mind. There is no stigma attached to a group simply out for a stroll; yet, with the common bond of understanding what it is like to experience mental illness, a healing environment is born.

9. **Mindfulness.** Mindfulness is being present, being in the moment. It saves us from ourselves, taking us away from regretting the past or worrying about the future. Examining the detail within leaves, the variation in colors, the contours and ridges of tree bark, and countless other aspects of the environment that might otherwise escape our conscious thought is an act of mindfulness. Exercising in greenspace while consciously being mindful of nature affords an opportunity to get outside your head.

### Exercising Mindfulness

In 1941, Yale professor, psychiatrist, and one-time president of the American Psychiatric Association Dr. Arthur H. Ruggles initiated a nature therapy program for mental health at Butler Hospital in Providence, Rhode Island. The initiative combined therapeutic walking with a conscious direction of thoughts to the natural world.

A study published in the *Journal of Environmental Psychology* in 2011 validates Ruggles's outside-the-box thinking, showing that the benefits of outdoor exercise can be enhanced by active cognitive consideration of the natural environment. Specifically, participants in one group were asked to be mindful of the environment, to make visualizations and inferences related to the natural world, to be aware of sounds, to actively seek out beauty, and to think about what they might change in the outdoor environment as they walked through it. The second group walked outdoors for the same allotted times; however, they were not instructed to be mindful of their surroundings. After two weeks, the psychological benefits of the outdoor exercise plus cognitive engagement were significantly higher versus walking without mindful instruction and certainly higher than no outdoor exercise at all—as with the third, control group.

10. **Exercise snacks.** It has become increasingly evident that for health, exercising in a traditional sense (working out once a day) may not be enough to offset otherwise sedentary behavior. In other words, you may do a morning jog for 30 minutes, but if you spend the rest of the day sitting on a chair in front of a screen, that 30 minutes of exercise is diluted. In fact, some research shows that it ultimately gets undone by the elevated health risks associated with sitting too long. The bottom line is move and move often. When you need a break, instead of reaching for a cookie, grab an exercise snack—get up from

your office chair, walk for a few minutes or do some stretching, and look outside the window to get a glimpse of nature. Even a small "fun size" piece of physical activity is a minor dose of exercise, and one that ultimately contributes to your brain health. Research has shown that the mental benefits of exercising in greenspace can be evident in as little as five minutes, even when exercising at a very light intensity.

## The Green Standard in Exercise

Green exercise has proven its worth. Outdoor exercise not only turns up the dial on intentions to stick with an exercise program but it specifically increases self-esteem and positive affect—key indicators that transform good intentions into action and initial bouts of exercise into regular physical activity. Combining all the brain benefits of exercise with the distinct mental benefits of immersion in greenspace—cognitive enhancing and mood-regulating benefits— magnifies them. Greenspace exercise should be considered a brain tonic, a therapeutic intervention that serves as a preventive agent warding off stress and its consequences, and one that can be reached for when the psychological seas are rough. Indeed, researchers have shown that the sedentary and those with mental distress have the most to gain from greenspace exercise. The ability of greenspace exercise to foster positive thoughts and decrease the negative ones associated with exercise can enhance the intention and motivation to stick with the plan and allow individuals to continue taking "the medicine." As it becomes evident that positive affect is the facilitator of exercise adherence, it seems obvious that the answer to the compliance problem may, at least to some degree, be found in green exercise. The end result is a fast-acting, low-cost intervention, open to all and devoid of side effects.

# Kingdom Animalia: The Last Stronghold of Nature on the Brain

*Man's machine-age technology has systematically
alienated him from nature, but possibly
his ancient friend, the animal, can prove
helpful... with a pet, most of us recreate
unconsciously the time long ago when we had
clear skies, wide-open spaces and an
unhurried existence.*

—Boris M. Levinson, PhD, 1972

Nature isn't just plants, trees, rocks, and water; it also encompasses the wild and domesticated animals that coexist with us. As with other elements of nature, human fascination with animals appears to be written deep into our genetic code. Studies show that we can rapidly identify animals in nature scenes—within a fraction of a second we can zero in on them. We are also more sensitive to changes in positioning of animals than other objects (such as vehicles) within an environment. Even infants visually process and categorize animals faster than they do nonanimal objects. The fact that we direct rapid attention to animals in an environment should not be surprising; after all, we have grown up with them for the last 2 million years, and for our survival it would obviously be necessary to instantaneously determine if we are being viewed as prey. Although we feared them as a source of danger, they also sustained us both as a source of nourishment and as an indicator of where water, edible plants, and other food sources might be. Put simply, it's served us well to pay attention to animals. It has also served us well to befriend a few of them. For at least the last 14,000 years, humans have had a special bond and mutually beneficial relationship with domesticated dogs—animals that provided protection, hunting and shepherding, and companionship. Cats have been domesticated for close to 10,000 years and although they don't have top-class shepherding skills and they are rarely seen being used by protective service agencies, they are the world's most popular pet.

In developed nations, the threat of wild animals in daily life has now been minimized, contact with the animals used for nourishment is basically nonexistent, and, with the advent of the produce section and the bottled water aisle in supermarkets, we no longer need animals to point the way to edible plants and water. And yet, dogs, cats, and a wide variety of other animals have been brought into human living quarters in staggering numbers. Despite our immersion in technology, we are still holding fast to our attraction to animals. Moreover, the pet explosion in the last 40 years may be due in part to our broad withdrawal from nature—pets provide the last stronghold of nature contact.

Since the introduction of screen gadgets and wireless devices in earnest over the last decade, the pet acquisition and care industry has more than doubled its market value. In 1998, the industry was worth US$23 billion; it has since grown to a staggering US$50-plus billion. The number of dogs in North America has far outpaced population growth: in the 1970s, there was a dog for every seven people; now there is a dog for every four people, and nearly a single pet for every man, woman, and child in North America. Numerous articles and editorials suggest that there may be a hint of narcissism in this increasing dog acquisition, with some pet owners viewing dogs as fashion accessories, emulating celebrity culture. The increase in spending isn't solely accounted for by a rise in pet ownership; there has also been a shift in the way we indulge our animal companions—pet day spas and hotels, acupuncture and massage, dietary supplements and expensive meal plans are no longer fringe options. We certainly are not casting judgment on this pattern: after 14,000 years of dedicated service to humans, maybe it is time that dogs received more than a bone with a bit of meat on it. Our view is one of positivity, and our suspicion, as others have contended before us, is that a rise in pet ownership meets a fundamental drive for nature contact in an increasingly synthetic world.

As we discuss in this chapter, the role of companion animals in the promotion of human health and survival is not restricted to the historical roles of the past—focused as they were on the hunting and protective skills of dogs and the rodent control by cats. On the contrary, research shows that domestic animals are as important to positive health as they have ever been. In fact, with the continued erosion of nature contact, animals take on a magnified role in the promotion of overall health, and mental health in particular.

## Get Us to the Green—Physical Benefits of Pet Ownership

In the mid-1970s, biologist Erika Friedmann and her colleagues began to examine the physiological changes induced by pets, as well as some of the health outcomes in large groups of pet owners. They showed, for example, that petting an animal could minimize stress on the blood circulatory system compared with other activities, including reading. However, it was their landmark study published in 1980 in *Public Health Reports* that caused the medical community to sit up and take notice. For this investigation they recruited patients who had recently been treated in a hospital for either a heart attack or angina and followed them for one year. The results showed that 28 percent of the individuals who did not have pets died within the year, whereas only 6 percent of the pet owners died during the same time frame. The difference was not merely due to the ability of dogs to get their owners out the door for some physical activity; even when dog owners were removed from the data, the protection afforded by pets still remained. Subsequent studies by other research teams have shown that pet ownership is associated with less frequent visits to health-care providers, less prescription medication use, and greater adherence to medical treatment programs.

While it's tempting to dismiss these associations as simply indicating that pet owners are generally a healthier lot to begin with, it is noteworthy that researchers have found general health and behaviors associated with health improve after the acquisition of a pet. In one specific study published in *Hypertension* in 2001, adults with high-stress jobs began blood-pressure medication therapy to address hypertension. They were randomized into one of two groups: those who received medication only and those who also acquired a cat or dog. When the researchers followed up with all participants six months later, they found that the cat and dog owners had lower blood pressure elevations subsequent to cognitive stress than the subjects who only took medication. Moreover, compared with baseline performance scores on stressful mental tasks, those in the pet acquisition group improved their accurate performance by almost 20 percent, whereas the medication-only group remained unchanged. Since cardiovascular disease and its mortality rate are highly linked to stress physiology, depressive mental outlook, anxiety, and lack of social support, researchers began to have a closer look at the ways in which companion animals influence physiology.

## Truly Man's Best Friend

Among all animals that provide human companionship and fascination, our dogs are most likely to get us off the couch and out into green. In Chapter 5 we discussed in detail the research on exercise and the brain, and the emerging notion that exercise in nature might be considered the "green standard" in the promotion of human health. For as long as it has been known that excess weight is a contributor to various diseases, dog acquisition has been prescribed by physicians as a way to reduce weight through promotion of physical activity.

Contemporary research has shown that dog ownership increases the odds of being a more physically active teenager or adult. Moreover, dogs can increase the likelihood that an owner will show up in greenspace, and dog owners do not see the predictable dip in winter walking found in nonowners. Having a dog is, of course, not an automatic inducer of physical activity; it simply increases the likelihood. For those who actually walk their dogs—versus sliding open the back door and letting the dog take care of business on its own—the odds of meeting guidelines for moderate to vigorous physical activity are significantly increased, and perhaps unsurprisingly, the odds of being obese are significantly decreased. (The back-door-opening, nonwalking dog owners are on a par with adults who do not own dogs in terms of physical activity and obesity rates.) However, the health benefits of dog ownership extend beyond physical activity per se, and we simply cannot discount that fact that dogs are not just a palpable piece of nature: they bring their human caregivers back full circle into the broad context of nature.

## Animals and Mental Health Care

The use of animals to prevent and treat mental illness dates back several centuries. Most experts point to the famous York Retreat in the United Kingdom, opened in 1796, as among the first institutions to specifically encourage interactions with nonthreatening animals, not merely as a distraction but as a way to actively "awaken the social and benevolent feelings" of the patients. Therapeutic walks were designed to pass through courts home to various small animals, including rabbits and birds, a practice that facilitated interaction and familiarity with the creatures. In addition, patients were encouraged to tend to plants and exercise within the expansive greenspace, referred to as "airing grounds." The York Retreat received good press on both sides of the Atlantic, and although it did not bring about the routine use of animals in mental health care, the policies did contribute to a shift in compassionate mental health care within institutional settings. York provided a clear example that there was an alternative to restraint and oppressive conditions.

Near the close of World War II, the United States military embraced the therapeutic value of animals when it converted a near-700-acre prep school in Pawling, N.Y., into a special rehabilitation center for ailing veterans. Half of the veterans were suffering from anxiety and mental anguish related to combat and stress reactions, referred to at the time under the soft term "operational fatigue." Working in cooperation with the Red Cross, local leaders of the Society for the Prevention of Cruelty to Animals and animal-loving donors, they initiated a Dog for Every Patient project. A 1945 *Newsweek* article summed up the mental health benefits of the canine companion program: "The dogs have been responsible for a minor miracle of such great curative value and of such simplicity that is a wonder it hadn't been thought of before . . . the time of convalescence has been cut immensely." The military also encouraged participation in nature study, contact with the soil through gardening and farming, and active participation in the care of a variety of animals. At Pawling there was a sign that specifically stated "Please Walk on the Grass!" Despite its reported success, this paradise, as it was known by those with operational fatigue, was short-lived, and in 1946, the same year that many of the glowing reports on the project were emerging, money was tight and the military surrendered the lease on the grounds.

Despite the attention Pawling received during its short tenure, it did little to spur a movement of further investigation related to companion animals and mental health. Post–World War II mental health was dominated by the emergence of miracle pills, including Miltown, a supposed antianxiety drug that was widely prescribed. Miltown, it turned out later in a scientific inquiry, was nothing more than a placebo that simply induced some noticeable side effects suggesting that it was "doing something."

While teams of scientists worked diligently to discover the next big chemical placebo, a lone voice called for a different line of inquiry.

In 1961, New York clinical psychologist Boris M. Levinson addressed the American Psychological Association's annual meeting, describing his experiences using a dog as a cotherapist. The response at the time was reported to be lukewarm, and indeed Levinson's contention that the presence of a dog facilitates initial dialogue was even ridiculed by some of his peers. Levinson, however, remained committed to researching and writing on the topic of the human-animal bond. As the years unfolded, ridicule turned into widespread support. It was a slow process—20 years in the making—and aided by some high-profile interviews in leading magazines, but by the 1980s, Levinson was speaking to packed auditoriums, and more importantly, he fostered a culture of scientific inquiry into the mental health benefits of animal contact. Along the way he sensed that, although the computer age was beginning to drive humans away from nature, we would turn to pets in order to grasp nature and create an inner sense of calm.

Levinson would be proved right. Studies have shown the benefit of animals (therapy dogs in particular) in patients with anxiety, irritability, and mood disturbances. They have been shown to improve mental outlook and overall quality of life, diminish aggression and hyperactivity, and improve energy levels. There is an abundance of research on social support—friends, family, and colleagues—providing a buffer against stress, anxiety, and depressive symptoms. Yet, although most dog and cat owners consider their pets part of the family, pets have never really been considered part of the true social support network in mental health. Given a new study published in 2011 in the *Journal of Personality and Social Psychology*, it might be time to reconsider this. The study reported that pets fulfill social connectivity needs, promote well-being, and provide an additional layer of social support on top of the circle of human support. Most telling was that a pet could stave off negative psychological reactions in a setting where the study participants were subjected to a social rejection experiment. As the researchers stated, "One's pet was every bit as effective as one's best friend" when it came to lending support and buffering the typical negativity of social rejection. Backing all of this up is a 2011 survey of over 2,000 adults that showed that pets owners were happier in general—and 60 percent of the pet owners surveyed attributed their increased personal happiness to having a pet.

## Strengthening the Case with Science

Despite anecdotal reports that companion animals play a role in positive mental health and despite their use in various health-care settings, the notion of pet therapy has largely remained off the radar of mainstream medicine. Scientific inquiry is the only way to evaluate the intuition surrounding the mental benefits of pets and, if confirmed, the only passage to widespread clinical acceptance.

In a clever 1991 experiment, researchers at the State University of New York had dog owners perform complex cognitive tasks in three settings: while alone, with a friend seated nearby, or with their own dog sitting in the vicinity (but not closer than three feet). Remarkably, the various physiological markers of stress reactivity were lowest when testing was conducted with the animal nearby. Furthermore, the results showed that the subjects performed significantly better on a stressful cognitive task with their pet nearby—even though their human friends had been told that the experiment was set up to evaluate social support and reactions to stress. (No such instructions were given to the dogs.)

Research from Virginia Commonwealth University shows that when health-care professionals interact with a friendly dog for as little as five minutes, they experience significant reductions in the stress hormone cortisol. When adult volunteers are subjected to stressful cognitive tasks, interaction with therapy dogs buffers the usual stress reaction and cortisol elevations. Given the destructive force of chronically elevated cortisol in a harried, stressful environment, an intervention that can lower stress hormones should be welcome for consideration. Even the simple act of petting a dog has been shown to reduce physiological markers of stress reactivity and improve immune system function. Research using sophisticated electroencephalograph (EEG) readings has shown that interacting with therapy dogs brings about changes in brain wave activity that are in line with states of mental relaxation.

A number of studies have shown that interacting with dogs can cause an increase in the production of oxytocin. Oxytocin, a hormone-like peptide produced in the brain, is in many ways the elixir of positive psychology. It has been shown to facilitate social bonding, prosocial behavior, and empathy; decrease stress; improve mental outlook; turn down the dial on activity in the fear centers of the brain; enhance a sense of security, trust, and pleasure; and lower the production of stress hormones. At present, international scientists are hard at work with synthetic oxytocin, investigating and patenting various means and delivery methods to boost oxytocin levels. In the meantime, interacting with animals can provide a lift to our own oxytocin levels, as well as those of the animals: petting dogs and laboratory animals caused a rise in both the subject's oxytocin levels and that of the animal.

This two-way street of oxytocin production may be at the heart of the human-animal bond, and given the direct social and personal health implications of oxytocin, it may provide physiological clues as to why pets promote mental health. It may also help explain why dogs work so well in counseling settings. Research has shown that psychotherapists are viewed more favorably when evaluated in the presence of a dog, and individuals report themselves as more likely to disclose deeply personal information when the psychotherapist is in the presence of a dog. Meanwhile, the administration of oxytocin increases the perception of trust in another, a factor that is at the very core of the psychotherapeutic alliance. Recently it was reported that the administration of oxytocin (versus placebo) made couples' conflict discussions more positive and reduced the production of stress hormones after conflict resolution sessions.

## Animal Interactions and Cognitive Performance

In 1902, Dr. Clifton F. Hodge of Clark University encouraged the introduction of small animals and plants into the classroom, referring to them as "the key to the door into knowledge." He suspected that animal observation and interaction would have far-reaching effects in cognitive development. Modern research supports his position. For example, in 2002, Japanese researchers showed that the simple act of keeping goldfish in early childhood seemed to expand knowledge of broader aspects of marine biology and enhance the ability of these children to draw analogies from their experiences with goldfish and apply them to other species and animals. Similar findings were reported by the same Japanese team when a group of 5-year-olds were studied. The children came from households containing either dogs, hamsters, or no animals, and the results once again showed that children with pets had a more expansive knowledge of animals overall and the ability to extend newly taught information related to dogs or hamsters and appropriately apply it to other animal species.

Although it would be easy to assume that the presence of animals might act as a cognitive distracter, bringing children and adults off task, the research findings related to mental performance show the opposite. In a series of recently published studies with children, Dr. Nancy Gee and colleagues from the State University of New York have shown that the presence of a dog can minimize errors on cognitive tasks, enhance memory performance, increase adherence to verbal instruction, and accelerate the pace of tasks involving motor skills—without any loss in accuracy. And as mentioned earlier, in a separate study from State University of New York researchers, when adult volunteers were subjected to stressful cognitive tests, they performed better in the presence of a dog than when they were alone or with a friend.

Recent studies have shown us that even in early infancy, children show higher degrees of eye fixations when observing images of animals in their natural settings than they do when looking at isolated animal images cut and pasted to a white background, and their reactions to real animals indicate a much higher degree of fascination compared with contact with animal toys. Pet exposure during the first six months of life brings about definite changes in the way infants cognitively process scenes with animals. Infants from households with pets appear more fascinated with animals, spending more time and attention on animal images when they are presented away from home in a laboratory setting. How these early experiences with animals and these differences in animal-related cognition shape the brain later in life remains a mystery, although it is becoming increasingly clear that experience with animals early in life leads to a more empathic brain later in life.

Like so much in nature, animals are inherently magnetic to humans; we pay them attention involuntarily, unlike the mundane tasks of our modern lives that demand concentrated, voluntary attention. When we are engaged with nature and its fascinating elements, eliminating (inhibiting) nonpertinent information requires minimal mental effort. Interacting with animals typically involves involuntary attention, provides us with a dose of fascination, and ultimately leads to a reduction of mental fatigue and a sense of cognitive restoration. Interactions with animals also foster positive thoughts, which can subsequently maximize cognitive performance and creativity. Given the ability of nonthreatening animals to reduce stress reactivity, thereby lowering the height of a major hurdle to cognitive performance, it's not surprising that animal interaction can lead to a sharper brain.

## Animals and Empathy

The potential for empathy is hard-wired in the normally functioning human brain. Yet, these neural pathways of empathy might be considered kindling in need of a match. Experience is, in many instances, the match that lights the fires of empathy. Because empathy involves the ability to cognitively and emotionally understand or apprehend the experience and emotions of another, it follows that experience dictates a fair degree of empathic response. For example, although all adults are capable of expressing great empathy for children, evidence suggests that parents express higher degrees than adults without children.

In the last decade, a number of studies have shown that pet ownership (of dogs in particular) in childhood is positively linked with empathy during the early years, and it is also predictive of subsequent empathy in adulthood. Importantly, pet ownership in childhood is not only associated with enhanced sensitivity to the distress of animals—this might be expected—but it also broadens human-directed empathic attitudes. In 2001, European scientist Vlasta Vizek Vidović evaluated 356 university students. She reported that pet ownership in childhood increases the odds that an individual will be drawn to adult work in the helping professions. The students who owned a pet in childhood also scored better on tests designed to evaluate prosocial behavior, including the willingness to make sacrifices for others and the environment, than those students without a childhood pet. Note that children can benefit from exposure to animals even outside of pet ownership per se. Both school-based interventions involving humane educational sessions regarding animals and the presence of a dog in a classroom for three months have been shown to foster empathy.

The higher an individual's empathic scores are in general, the more that person cares about the welfare of animals. Our allegiance to our animal friends seems to exist on a continuum: we show the highest levels of empathic concern for mammals, the creatures most like us, then for birds and other members of the animal kingdom. (Interestingly, research has shown that mammals and birds are capable of empathy for their own kind. As we write, the first studies are attempting to confirm what countless dog owners have long claimed: dogs, by virtue of their 14,000-plus year contact with humans, appear to show true empathic concern for humans.) With the understanding that empathy bonds us to each other, the inference of such research is that human-animal interactions can make the world a better place. So instead of stroking the keyboard or rubbing the belly of your smartphone screen, you—and the world—will be better served by petting your dog (or your goldfish).

## Aqua Friends

> A man can sit for hours before an aquarium and stare into it as into the flames of an open fire or the rushing waters of a torrent. All conscious thought is happily lost in this state of apparent vacancy, and yet, in these hours of idleness, one learns essential truths about the macrocosm and the microcosm.
>
> —*Nobel laureate Konrad Lorenz, 1952*

In the mid-1800s, not long after the technology allowed for them, the popularity of public aquariums blossomed. They were described at the time, by leading authorities William R. Hughes and James Shirley Hibberd, as being ideal "as a relief and mental refreshment for those in crowded courts for whom the sea is but a name!" and "aids in the cultivation of kindness and the enlargement of general knowledge." Although aquarium fish are probably not the first pets that come to mind when we think about companion animals, they are still a source of wonder, and after more than 150 years, the aquarium industry remains in the business of mental refreshment. In 1979, Boris M. Levinson reported in *Psychological Reports* that aquariums in the offices of mental health providers may induce relaxation and enhance dialogue in the therapeutic sessions. Following publication of this report, separate groups of researchers confirmed the ability of office aquariums to reduce anxiety and improve objective markers of stress. Contemplation of an aquarium was reported to have an edge in stress reduction over medical hypnosis or contemplation of a nature poster of a mountain waterfall.

In the last few years, the acquisition of high-end home aquariums, particularly by adult men, has grown by leaps and bounds. No one is quite sure what is driving the resurgence of aquariums over the last decade. As British writer Edward Docx wrote eloquently in a 2011 *Prospect* magazine article, "Some cite Disney's 2003

> film *Finding Nemo* as the moment when aquariums started coming back ... some say bling, some say gadgets, some say calm and some say creation. Others speculate that it's because aquariums have everything: art, science, nature."

## Animal Goggles

Most people are familiar with the term "beer goggles," a phenomenon whereby members of the opposite sex increase in attractiveness in direct proportion to the amount of alcohol the beholder has consumed. Australian psychologists made international headlines in 2011 when they confirmed this in natural settings (the habitats of university students: campus pubs and parties). But altering the attractiveness of individuals and environments through beer goggles has many downsides, not the least of which are increased risk taking and hangovers. Luckily, animals can also change our view of the world—without the negative effects of alcohol. Studies show that when animals are in an environment, everything looks better, including people.

In 1981, psychologist Randall Lockwood, now a senior vice-president at the American Society for the Prevention of Cruelty to Animals, presented the first research findings on the extent to which animals might influence environmental perceptions. Adult volunteers were asked to examine various illustrated scenes involving ambiguous situations involving one or two humans. The volunteers reviewed the scenes in fairly rapid fashion (a minute or two per scene). They also viewed an identical set of scenes with just a single variable altered: an animal (cat, dog, or bird) had been added as an outlier in the scene. For example, in one scene a child appears to have been just tucked into bed by an adoring mother. The companion scene was identical except a cat was curled up at the end of the bed. Volunteers rated the scenes that included animals more positively and identified the humans depicted in these scenes as more likeable, friendly, happy, confident, and less stressed than those in scenes where there was no animal. Other studies would soon follow, with researchers reporting that when subjects viewed adults photographed with a companion dog, they were rated as more stylish, active, relaxed, and happy. More recently, researchers presented undergraduate volunteers with various photographs of university professors' offices, some of which contained a companion animal. Even though the professors were not present in any of the photographs, offices with a dog were perceived to belong to a friendly professor, and rooms containing a cat were thought to be occupied by professors who were less harried. Combined, these findings show that we perceive an adult with an animal as safe and approachable.

In real-world settings, dogs significantly increase the likelihood of contact between a dog walker and stranger, with research showing this is especially true when the dog is being walked in greenspace. Dogs, therefore, are social facilitators. And it's not just dogs that make us look cool: when a sample of 542 adults viewed photographs of males, first posed with a cat and then with a dog, subjects rated the men as nicer and more stylish when they posed with the cat.

Using pets as a sort of icebreaker to short-circuit some of the barriers to social communication in public settings has obvious benefits, and these benefits can be magnified in the mental-health-care realm. As mentioned, a pet in the room of a psychotherapist can positively influence the confidence ratings of potential patients. In 2006, University of Toronto psychologist Margaret Schneider examined the "dog in the room" phenomenon and had 85 adults view videotapes of psychotherapists describing their work and expertise. The altered variable, as you have probably guessed, was the presence or absence of a dog, in this case a golden retriever lying quietly on the floor. Participants viewed the psychotherapists much more favorably if a dog was in the room during the videotaped session, scoring them higher on the well-established Counselor Rating Form and its specific "trustworthy" scale. Study participants were also more willing to disclose personal information to the psychotherapists with a dog in the room. Since positivity, trust, and willingness to disclose personal thoughts and feelings are at the very heart of the psychotherapeutic alliance, the results have broad implications. Often the initial sessions with mental health professionals are the most difficult for patients—anxiety runs high—therefore, even a small amount of stress reduction in these early treatment efforts can pay massive dividends.

---

### A Note of Caution

Despite spending an entire chapter positioning companion animals as a bridge to the natural world, we must also acknowledge that keeping a pet is not for everyone, and not every animal is suitable to become a pet. Visiting the American Society for the Prevention of Cruelty to Animals (ASPCA) or the Humane Society of Canada's website will make this fact abundantly clear. The ASPCA (and its Canadian counterparts) recognizes in its policy statement that the human-animal bond is undeniable and that careful pet maintenance is of value to the animal and the human. However, in order for this mutual benefit to be maintained, there must be a serious commitment on the part of the human to meet the criteria for responsible care.

Setting aside the very serious issues of puppy mills, exotic pets, dog fighting, animal hoarding, show-biz animals, and other grave concerns, it is not uncommon for otherwise well-meaning individuals to get in over their heads with pet acquisition. Responsible pet care, even at its most basic level, involves an investment in time, energy, and money. Given the research we have discussed in this chapter—the benefits related to stress, health of mind and body, and mental acuity—the pet owner will ultimately receive all of his or her investments back, and then some. However, it would be inappropriate for us to advocate pet prescriptions without acknowledging that crowded shelters translate into more than 4 million cats and dogs being put down every year in North America—an animal every eight seconds. So please carefully consider the level of responsibility required to properly care for your pet of choice and ensure it will fit into your lifestyle *before* you acquire it.

---

## The Canaries in Our Coal Mine

In recent history, animals, much like plants, have been a sad barometer of human environmental exploitation and pollution. There are multiple examples where the loss and early mortality of small animals—amphibians, reptiles, birds, fish, and mammals—have been discovered to be a result of exposure to even low-level environmental contaminants. Astute veterinarians have noticed clusters of increased domestic pet mortality and, while working with other scientists, have traced the diminished longevity to local environmental contamination. This area of research, known generally as wildlife toxicology (although it does include domestic pets), has always been in the business of playing catch-up. Industry introduces chemicals for widespread application (such as aerial pesticide use and polychlorinated biphenyls or PCBs in the 1920s and 1930s), and society does not seriously consider the effect on wildlife until decades later. The 1962 publication of Rachel Carson's book *Silent Spring* was, among other things, a wake-up call about the effects of pesticides on human and nonhuman animals. Although pesticides had been in use for decades before Carson's book, the project was inspired by a 1958 letter published in the *Boston Herald* regarding the reported loss of birds, as well as grasshoppers, bees, and other insects, as a result of DDT-spraying practices. While *Silent Spring* galvanized an environmental movement and changed laws governing environmental contaminants, it would be naive to think that Kingdom Animalia is now safe. On the contrary, more than half a century post–*Silent Spring*, chemicals such as flame retardants are showing up in increasingly high amounts in the eggs of wild birds, while the numbers of amphibians, bats, bees, butterflies, beetles, and other insects are declining en masse. It is a global problem on a colossal scale. Declines in all of the aforementioned creatures, the most vulnerable in our animal world, hit the fast lane in the last two decades—and this should tell us that something in our environment has dramatically changed.

## Animals Tangled Up in Wireless Signals?

One factor that has changed our living environment in unfathomable ways is the massive global introduction of wireless communication. Consider that the total number of wireless subscribers in the United States has risen from 4.3 million in 1990 to some 300 million today. More importantly, though, are the mobile phone towers and semi-disguised antennas embedded in the environment—4,800 in 1990 have been transformed into an incredible 250,000-plus towers, with an ever-increasing number springing up like dandelions on a lawn. For years, scientists told us not to worry: wireless phones are innocuous because they do not cause heat damage to the tissue (such as the human brain) close to exposure sites in the way that a microwave oven can. The message was simple: no heat (thermal changes), no problem. This simple message has, however, been collapsing like a house of cards. Researchers have now shown that electromagnetic radiation in the wireless range (900 to 1800 MHz) is well capable of causing damage to various cells, alter plant growth, and change animal behavior by means other than heat (i.e., nonthermal mechanisms). As researchers, including the World Health Organization expert panel, grapple with the extent to which wireless communication devices might impact human health, it is not our intent to transform this book into a diatribe against mobile phones. Rather, our concern in the current context is the influence of electromagnetic radiation in the wireless range on the sensitive members of the Kingdom Animalia and the plant world in which they reside.

In the late 1950s, several years before *Silent Spring* was published, accumulating data began to suggest that the introduction of human-made radio waves was not without consequence to the growth, development, health, and behavior of animals and plants. Even individuals who help put radio broadcasting on the map—including writer and publisher Hugo Gernsback—stated that expansion of terrestrial radio-wave production was not without peril. Plants, animals, and the human animal grew together over the years under the constant influence of gravity and electromagnetic forces. With wireless on the horizon, distinguished New York engineer Henry L. Logan warned in 1973 that "the technological age of the twentieth century represents the first total threat to man, because it changes the rules of survival as he has known them up to now, by changing his immediate environment—the basic electromagnetic and electrostatic fields in which he is immersed! Up to now, man has only had to contend with the natural fields to which he adapted . . ."

Scientists are still only just scratching the surface as to the extent to which plants respond to the environmental radiation via their own electrochemical signaling, and emerging research is showing the ways in which animals—from ants to loggerhead sea turtles—use electromagnetic forces to navigate, migrate, and nest. There is far more unknown about electromagnetic forces on animals than there is known, yet that has not stopped the tide of wireless radiation served up in the name of profits and progress.

In looking at wildlife toxicology research over the last several decades, it is becoming increasingly clear that in many cases it is the accumulation of various environmental pollutants and stressors, rather than a single agent, that poses the greatest threat to the natural world. And herein might be the real problem of electromagnetic pollution. For example, research has shown that electromagnetic radiation in the wireless device range can increase the permeability of the otherwise tight network of blood vessels around the brain of mammals (i.e., it makes the blood-brain barrier more porous). What does this mean in a practical sense? Since it is the primary function of the blood-brain barrier to keep undesirable material (think environmental contaminants) out of the brain, consider then how detrimental a compromised blood-brain barrier via electromagnetic radiation might be if an animal of any sort is exposed to pesticides. In order to prevent a decline in populations, insects and other animals must have full capacity to reproduce, yet here again research has shown that exposure to electromagnetic radiation in the wireless device range can compromise insect reproduction. It can also compromise normal nesting habits and 24-hour circadian rhythms, and perhaps most importantly, it can have a detrimental effect on the immune system.

Biologist Alfonso Balmori has summarized dozens of recent studies on electromagnetic pollution and animal life—his work was published in 2009 in the prestigious peer-reviewed journal *Pathophysiology* under the title "Electromagnetic pollution from phone masts: Effects on wildlife." Any individual who claims to care about the environment and its animals, scientists and nonscientists alike, should read and reread this work. Even more recently, in a two-month study, he has shown that in real-world urban settings, mobile phone towers increase the mortality of tadpoles in their vicinity—90 percent of them never make the transition from tadpole to a happy frog. Meanwhile, as we go to press, Marie-Claire Cammaerts and colleagues from the Université Libre de Bruxelles, Belgium have published research showing that electromagnetic radiation in the wireless range is detrimental to the ability of ants to secure food using environmental cues. Consider that more than 1 million bats have died in North America over the last few years, reportedly due to a fungus-causing "white nose syndrome." Yet, the suspect fungus has been around bats for a long time, so the real question is why are bats dying off en masse from a fungus that is not novel? What is wrong with their immune system? Why are they losing the battle against this fungal agent? Pesticide exposure to bees is not new, so, again, the real question is why are they dying off en masse from what appears to be only very low levels of pesticide accumulation?

The mass introduction of electromagnetic radiation is not a smoking gun in the case of vulnerable animal decline, and the sensational media reports such as "Mobile phones killing bees" are sort of like the "Google is making us smarter" headlines—they are not in line with what has been discovered, at least not yet. However, there is enough research to show that, at the very least, human-manufactured electromagnetic radiation is a source of stress to animals and may therefore be one piece of the puzzle. If we serve up electromagnetic radiation together with other sources of environmental stress, perhaps a chaser of pesticides—or any other more widely recognized environmental contaminant—we just might have a lethal cocktail. For now, to put it in its most simple terms, there is no convincing evidence that our massive introduction of electromagnetic radiation is *not* a player in the loss of biodiversity.

In chasing our profit-driven technology, humans don't exactly have an amazing track record when it comes to safeguarding the animals of the natural world, and quite possibly our own species welfare as well. If there is even an ounce of scientific credibility in these early studies on electromagnetic pollution and wildlife, then we have on our hands a more inconvenient truth than we could have ever imagined. Clearly, it will be difficult to ask who among us will turn off their wireless devices and protest Wi-Fi rollouts because they interfere with the survival of frogs, birds, and bees, among other insects. Will we really care enough if the environmental variable—that is, the mobile phone—is basically part of the human appendage, something so personal to us? Or will we sweep *that* research under the rug, content in the knowledge that we recycle and use canvas instead of plastic? The ethical dilemmas for the conscientious, for those most concerned about the ethical treatment of all animals, would be tremendous. Let's hope Dr. Balmori and his colleagues are all wrong on this.

## Moving Forward

Almost 40 years ago, clinical psychologist and pet therapy expert Boris M. Levinson was asked to speculate on what the human-pet world might look like in the year 2000 and beyond. Levinson turned out to be quite the soothsayer, predicting an explosion in pet acquisition thanks to the computer-driven, technological world. In January 1974, he said: "Suffering from even greater feelings of alienation than those which are already attacking our emotional health, future man will be compelled to turn to nature and the animal world to recapture some sense of unity with a world that otherwise will seem chaotic and meaningless . . . in the year 2000 pets will become a very important safety valve in a sick society."

Levinson's future has arrived. Pets appear to be every bit the safety valve that Levinson was predicting, and they do, in an increasingly plastic world, provide a sense of unity with nature. Levinson already knew from his experiences in the early 1960s that companion animals could be a form of psychotherapeutic medicine. He had the foresight to recognize that in the cybernetic future world, humans were going to be seeking a whole lot more of that particular medicine. With an accumulation of various studies, we can today recognize at least some of the value inherent in the human–companion animal connection. The notion of walking into a pet store and acquiring a pet as a form of self-medication is becoming more widely accepted, even endorsed, by health experts in the mainstream. The idea that caring for and interacting with a companion animal is akin to acquiring a prescription for a combined antianxiety and antidepressant drug is no longer laughable to those concerned with scientific evidence.

Research shows that almost 60 percent of pet owners would choose their pet as the single companion if they were stranded on a desert island. This sort of fantasy question isn't frivolous; it taps into the depths of the human-animal bond, and the answers to it underscore how important animals are to our mental health and survival. If the majority of adults choose an animal companion over family and friends in an imagined scenario of a fight for survival, we really begin to see a clear picture of what animals mean to us in today's society. However, we must also give serious consideration to how responsible pet care fits into the context of global animal welfare and biodiversity. Recently, this has become an area of passionate debate. Placing the rights of animals we cherish on a higher plane than their nondomesticated counterparts is a murky discussion that requires some cool-headed clarity. For example, researchers were recently surprised by the extent to which the global pet-food market is placing a burden on small wild-caught forage fish. Some 5.5 million metric tons of small wild fish are being consumed by pets—these are fish that are otherwise essential for seabirds, marine mammals, and larger predator fish. Specifically, research shows that a single domestic cat consumes almost twice as much fish than does the average North American human over the course of a year. Obviously, we should continue to feed our companion animals well; the message is that we should look for sustainable sources of protein and essential fats for our friends, sources that allow all members of the food chain to grow and thrive.

Similar debates are ongoing between bird conservation groups and cat owners. Wild bird advocates suggest that the overpopulation of domestic cats that are allowed outdoors or abandoned by irresponsible owners is in part responsible for the loss of millions of birds and small mammals, and an overall reduction in biodiversity. This is not a new debate. A 1916 report to the Massachusetts State Board of Agriculture referred to the free-roaming domestic cat as a "killer of wildlife"—what has changed in the last century is the urgency and seriousness with which we must address these issues. Interestingly, Levinson also warned some 40 years ago that in the year 2000 and beyond, "there will be increasing emphasis on living now—on the immediate experience—and less and less postponement of current pleasures for some future good." We are optimistic that prescriptions for pets will be viewed in the context of the future good of all animals and the biodiversity of the planet.

# Practical Nature Interventions: Horticultural and Wilderness Therapies

*There is no more healthful recreation for mind or body than gardening in all its branches, and it may be added that there is no recreation which will more thoroughly satisfy the inborn longing for the beautiful and the love of natural things. All who believe that there is a higher part of our nature that is worth cultivating will recognize the aesthetic side of gardening as one of its most beautiful influences.*

—Editors of *Scientific American*, 1897

*Closely allied with this task of developing inner resources of play and recreation is the role of camp in kindling the imagination, releasing fresh impulses, expanding and refining the emotions, and stimulating aesthetic appreciations and attitudes.*

—Hedley Dimock and Charles Hendry in *Camping and Character*, 1929

In the previous chapter, we discussed some of the encouraging findings of animal-assisted therapies, specific interventions using pets as a way to enhance mental well-being and stress resiliency. Here we continue with a closer look at two additional forms of nature-based therapies—horticultural (gardening) and wilderness (adventure-nature immersion)—examining the ways in which these therapies can help the brain. To be clear, legitimate horticultural and wilderness therapies are professionally operated by specially trained individuals, and they represent an organized extension of nature contact familiar to most of us. Outside of organized interventions, there are multiple brain benefits to simply toiling in the garden, to making contact with the earth, or roughing it in some challenging natural locales.

## Historical Aspects of Gardening for Mental Health

Humans have long been fascinated with a tiny seed's ability to develop, grow, and flourish into a source of sustenance. When cultivation techniques were established several thousand years ago, ancient Egyptians, for example, began to garden for reasons extending beyond the creation of food. Those who had the means, planted orderly gardens of ornamental flowers, shrubs, and trees for aesthetic beauty, privacy, and protection from the elements. Beyond the endgame itself—the functionality and aesthetics of fully mature plants—there was, and still is, a pleasure associated with the process of gardening: the inherent hope, challenge, fascination, and sense of purpose associated with nurturing life, all apparent in the mind of the gardener.

By the mid-1800s, physicians often promoted gardening as a mental relaxant. It was thought by the physicians of the time that the fresh air, exercise, and opportunity for contemplation provided by gardening could limit the need for frequent medical consultations. This thinking spurred the development of gardening programs within mental-health-care institutions. In 1843, Thomas S. Kirkbride, a noted physician and gardening advocate from Pennsylvania, set up a unique mental health institution that offered patients the opportunity to tend surrounding gardens and farmland. Kirkbride's vision, one that "presupposes a knowledge of the fact, that air was made for breathing, and that beauty of scenery is not unworthy of consideration in an asylum for the insane," was part of a broad effort to provide moral and compassionate treatment to those with mental health disorders. In the years that followed, Kirkbride became widely recognized for drawing up mandates on the design of mental health institutions, which included specific allocation for adjoining land for gardening and cultivation. Kirkbride stated that the gardens were "necessary appendages" and "can scarcely fail to prove exceedingly valuable, by contributing to the comfort, happiness, and restoration of many patients, as well as for the convenience and profit resulting from the abundant supplies of fresh vegetables derived from them."

By the early 1900s, gardening had become to some degree a mainstream activity broadly encouraged by directors of mental health institutions. In addition to the therapeutic value of gardening itself, patients in some institutions established hothouses and set up the flowering plants so that they were visible from inside the buildings, referring to them as "eye pastures" for mental health. However, the utility of gardening as a form of mental health therapy for shell-shocked soldiers established the budding profession of horticultural therapy.

In 1918, at the close of World War I, the U.S. military initiated gardening programs as adjunctive care for soldiers with shell shock (an early name for modern-day post-traumatic stress disorder). Guidance on the growth of vegetables and aromatic flowering plants, as well as artistic landscape gardening—so-called garden therapy—soon became the work of specially trained therapists under the auspices of occupational therapy.

Within the next decade, occupational therapy programs began offering specific horticultural therapy classes to prepare students for work in hospitals and mental health settings. And as early as 1929, "horticultural therapist for hospitals" was officially listed as a vocation, with competitive civil service positions offered within U.S. Veterans Bureau institutions. The outbreak of World War II created another enormous demand for mental-health-care services among military personnel. Once again, the mental health profession enlisted garden therapy as a critical means of assisting in rehabilitation. Both public and private funding in support of this effort, as well as its reported successes, helped to solidify horticultural therapy as a profession, with tremendous potential for advancement.

## From Anecdote to Scientific Inquiry

The value of horticultural therapy programs in military hospitals was not lost on civilian psychologists, psychiatrists, or mainstream mental-health-care experts. In the decades following World War II, select psychologists and other mental-health-care advocates continued to discuss the benefits of horticultural therapy and to encourage its expansion into more broad avenues of mental health care. However, although broad claims of success are interesting, for a developing profession to be taken seriously in contemporary health care, it needs to be supported by scientific inquiry.

This inquiry began in the 1970s, when Dr. Rachel Kaplan of the University of Michigan examined why healthy adults are drawn to gardening—what do they get out of the activity? Using psychological scales, the initial results showed that gardening provides a sense of fascination, a key contributor to involuntary attention and cognitive restoration. In addition, subjects gave high ratings to the sensory benefits of tilling and growing and to the opportunity for quiet and feelings of peacefulness and tranquility. The researchers also observed that gardeners reported a greater affinity with nature compared with nongardeners. Engagement with nature almost inevitably leads to more concern for nature.

These initial scientific investigations led to additional inquiry and, over the years, results have shown that horticultural programs can help improve motivation, communication, grief processing, depressive thoughts, anxiety, sleep, psychosocial skills, self-esteem, stress reduction, and overall psychological well-being. Recent studies examining the power of horticultural therapy in people with clinical depression demonstrate just how powerfully working with soil and plants can improve mental outlook.

In 2009, researchers at the Norwegian University of Life Sciences set up a 12-week therapeutic horticulture intervention that had participants sowing, germinating, potting, planting, rooting, cultivating, and cutting vegetables and flowers. Beyond merely tilling the soil, the participants, all of whom had moderate-heading-toward-severe depression, also indulged in usual gardener behavior—walking around their garden patch and sitting nearby and admiring it, while also looking for animal life, including butter-flies and other insects. All told, they gardened twice a week for three hours a session. Their depression scores improved significantly after the intervention. Additional psychological scales revealed a more detailed story: the degree of fascination reported by an individual gardener was the strongest predictor of improvement in depres-sion. Engendering fascination can help short-circuit depression's debilitating cycle of rumination—the negative thoughts that seem to run on a continuous loop. Three months after the researchers discontinued the horticultural intervention, the subject's depres-sion scores remained significantly lower than they had been before the start of the study, hinting at potential long-term benefits from a relatively short-term, low-cost intervention.

A similar 12-week study with similar design was published in 2010 in the *Journal of Advanced Nursing.* The results of the therapeutic horticulture program were on a par with cognitive behavioral therapy and medications, significantly improving scores of depression. Again, it was the improvement in cognitive focus associated with garden-ing that predicted improvement in depressive symptoms. This study showed an association between gardening and a reduction in brood-ing, lending further support to the notion that horticultural therapy activates specific brain pathways while disengaging internal rumina-tion. Building on this work, two separate studies published in 2011, one from Dalhousie University in Canada and the other from the Norwegian University of Life Sciences, indicate that gardening pro-vides a sense of purpose and meaning in life. Providing meaning and purpose may be one of the important contributions to the clinical value in depressive disorders and stress reduction in other chronic diseases associated with high risk of depression.

## Gardening, Physical Activity, and Stress Hormones

> *There is health in the garden. But because one has to dig for it, some persons prefer to keep on enjoying their old miserableness day after day and year after year . . . But those who are willing to exert themselves in an effort to get back the tone that life has lost to a considerable extent will find that work in the garden is a better tonic than our doctors have a record of in their pharmacopoeia.*
>
> —Eben E. Rexford, 1916

In the last few years, researchers have also looked at some of the physiological changes induced by the activity of gardening itself. Although many wouldn't consider it exercise, gardening is indeed a form of physical activity. Gardening maintains muscle strength and physical health through the aging process. Studies published in *HortTechnology* and *Acta Horticulturae* in 2008 and 2004 respectively have shown that gardening can be quite significant exercise. For example, 30 minutes of setting up, planting, and watering a flower bed was found to be the metabolic equivalent of a pickup game of basketball over the same duration. Obviously, gardening can, like any form of physical activity, vary in its intensity. Yet, for the average healthy adult, performing typical gardening activities over the course of 30 minutes is classified as a moderate-intensity physical activity, one that enables the individual to meet general physical activity recommendations. Even more encouraging is that, when people engage in gardening activities, they tend to do so for more than 30 minutes—combined data from the American Time Use Survey and the U.S. National Health and Nutrition Examination Survey show that the average time spent gardening is over 52 minutes. By way of comparison, the same surveys indicate that leisure walkers or treadmill users spend less than 30 minutes walking or using a treadmill.

Recently, researchers have begun to look at the effect of gardening on the stress hormone cascade. In an intriguing study published in a 2011 issue of the *Journal of Health Psychology*, researchers intentionally induced mental stress in adult gardeners via a complex cognitive computer task, after which the subjects either gardened outdoors or read from any one of a variety of popular magazines. In line with expectations, the stressful mental task elevated stress hormone levels and lowered positive mood states in the volunteers. Perhaps unsurprisingly to those of you with green thumbs, gardening reduced the stress hormone cortisol significantly more than reading did, and post-activity positive mood ratings were significantly higher in the gardening group—the higher the positive mental outlook post-gardening, the lower the cortisol levels.

In a 2010 German "Successful Aging and the Effect of Physical Activity" study, participants provided real-time data related to what they were up to and how they felt at a given moment. Collecting real-time data while subjects go about their regular routines (a technique known as ecological momentary assessment) increases the reliability of the reported data because it is superior to subjects' memory recall. Based on almost 2,000 real-time measurement points provided to investigators, gardening emerged as a physical activity that promotes a sense of contentment and calm, while at the same time increasing energy levels.

In a 1948 article in *Hygeia,* an official publication of the American Medical Association, it was stated that "the chief benefits of gardening as therapy lie in the dim, almost uncharted area of our emotions." It was predicted that the psychological distress of contemporary society would place increasing demands on physician time and resources and that, in the future, gardening would become a formal and routine prescription provided to psychologically stressed patients in general practice—the author provided a somewhat humorous example script: "Take 500 sq. ft. of ground, once daily—for external use only"—and went on to state that the "grateful patient will get his prescription filled, not at the local drugstore, but at the vacant corner lot, in a suburban development, or on a half-acre subdivision." Only one-half of the prediction has come true: the increasing influence of psychological stress in medical care and time constraints faced by physicians in the 21st century is certainly a reality. However, more than a half century later, modern prescriptions are dominated by drugs for anxious days and sleepless nights. Research shows that those with the highest levels of day-to-day stress have the most to gain from health-care provider recommendations for nature contact; yet, without the formal advice, they are reluctant to take action.

The *Hygeia* prediction for gardening prescriptions *should* be a reality by now. Gardening is one-part relaxant and one-part energizer, and it promotes health and happiness. And fortunately, the options for gardening are plentiful. One need not be a property owner to till a small plot of soil—rooftop gardens (so-called high-rise horticulture) and community or personal allotment gardens afford access to those without their own yard. In addition, many local botanical gardens in North American cities now offer supervised horticultural therapy programs for groups and individuals. And for those requiring formal assistance and follow-up from an allied health professional, trained horticultural therapists are at the ready for patient supervision and communicating with physicians.

---

### Community Gardens—Cultivating Nature in the City

Over 100 years ago, as metropolitan areas expanded in earnest, community gardens began to spring up out of vacant lots—the movement was initially called vacant lot gardening. Mostly, the lot landowners and city officials didn't object, as long as the gardeners surrendered the land if it was to be sold or developed. Organizations, such as New York's Vacant Lot Gardening Association, run by writer and attorney Bolton Hall, would legally make arrangements with

---

owners to utilize the lots and designate them for use by the unemployed or underprivileged. The vacant lot gardens became a highly successful way to, as one writer in *Technical World* stated in 1910, "bring nature back to our cities."

A century later, modern-day community gardens are alive and well, many of them continuing to serve individuals and families with socioeconomic, and therefore health, disparities. Access to nature in the form of parks and greenspace has been shown to be an equalizer of socioeconomic-related health disparity. Community gardens have the potential to amplify these benefits because the health-associated benefits of the gardens go beyond "seeing green" per se. From San Diego to Toronto, community gardens have been shown to increase access to healthy produce and enhance overall quality of nutritional intake, physical activity, mental health, social cohesion, local ecology, and sustainability. As psychologists Heather Okvat and Alex Zautra suggest, community gardens are the path to individual, community, and environmental resilience.

## Soil, Its Beneficial Bacteria, and the Brain

*With the simple exercise of a little prudent oversight,*
*the soil never did a child any harm . . . far richer is*
*what it gives than takes away. Far better are dollars*
*spent on children's clothes than pennies given to*
*doctors . . . every breath of leaf and soil makes finest*
*fibre, every moment gives pure and healthful delight.*
*The soil is the child's best friend.*
—"The Child's Dearest Playmate," Louisa Knapp, editor,
*Ladies' Home Journal,* 1898

*But if you are really elect in the ranks of*
*gardeners . . . you know what actual contact*

*with the soil and the things that grow therein means*
*in the way of mental and physical rejuvenation.*
—"Why Do People Garden?" Richardson Wright, editor,
*House and Garden,* 1918

Today, with assistance from marketers in the business of selling us antibacterial wipes, sprays, gels, soaps, and liquids, Western society has been scared into believing the overexaggerated notion that everything is "dirty." Broadly, all bacteria have been painted with the same brush, and that brush dictates that bacteria are bad. But not all bacteria are bad. Some of the bacteria found in soil and fermented foods can be good for us, and may even have a positive influence on our mental outlook. The roots of the connection between soil bacteria and mental health go back a century.

Elie Metchnikoff, winner of the Nobel Prize in Medicine in 1908, made a novel and remarkable claim that created a stir among microbiologists and scientists in general. He suggested that not only were the majority of bacteria residing in and passing through the gastrointestinal tract harmless but, indeed, some of them might actually be health-promoting. In his 1908 book, *The Prolongation of Life,* he noted the incredible longevity of Bulgarians and other Europeans at that time. He isolated a bacteria found in high amounts in the fermented foods consumed in these regions—*Bacillus bulgaricus,* later called *Lactobacillus bulgaricus,* and fed it to mice in an experimental setting. The mice that were given the bacteria lived significantly longer than the control mice—those not given the bacteria. He theorized that these beneficial bacteria were offsetting the production of toxins produced by other, potentially harmful, gastrointestinal intestinal bacteria.

While Metchnikoff focused on aging and longevity, some physicians thought the bacteria might offer potential benefit to mental health. In 1910, Dr. George Porter Phillips reported that orally administered *Lactobacillus bulgaricus* bacteria improved depressive symptoms in adults with melancholia. Before long, *Lactobacillus* yogurts and beverages were being marketed as mental tonics. What was little appreciated, and remains so today, was that *Lactobacillus bulgaricus* occurs naturally in soil, which scientists at the University of Chicago reported in 1909. The implication was that it would be fairly simple for gardeners to make incidental contact with healthy *Lactobacillus* while tilling the soil. Despite the early enthusiasm, interest in *Lactobacillus* for mental health and longevity waned, and by the mid-1930s it was off the radar, and would remain so for decades.

The *Lactobacillus*-mood story was quiet until it was unearthed in a scientific hypothesis paper in 2003. Our colleagues from the University of Toronto and McMaster University in Canada provided an updated theory supposing that *Lactobacillus* and its probiotic (life-promoting) partner genera *Bifidobacteria* could influence human mood and cognition. What had changed in the preceding few years were the new discoveries that these bacteria can reduce body-wide inflammation and oxidative stress. As we discussed in earlier chapters, the elevation of inflammatory chemicals called cytokines can cause depression, anxiety, and cognitive brain fog in healthy adults. Also newly discovered was that even miniscule levels of microbes passing through the intestinal tract could potentially influence mood by direct communication with the central nervous system via nerves connected to the gastrointestinal tract.

Additional clinical studies, published in 2009 and 2011, showed that orally consumed *Lactobacillus* and *Bifidobacteria* could improve mood, decrease anxiety, and improve cognitive functioning in adults. Recent experimental studies in animals show that when these bacteria are orally administered to animals that are under stress, the level of stress hormones in the brain is reduced, and the bacteria have a beneficial effect on the mood- and fear-regulating neurotransmitters in various parts of the brain. Through mechanisms that remain unclear, the beneficial bacteria inhibit the enzymes that otherwise break down mood-regulating neurotransmitters, and they maintain levels of the "miracle grow" nerve growth factor we discussed previously—brain-derived neurotrophic factor (BDNF), the chemical responsible for healthy nerve cell maintenance. Moreover, *Bifidobacteria* added to animal food increases brain omega-3 fatty acid levels and blood levels of tryptophan. Tryptophan is a vital amino acid required for the manufacture of the "feel good" chemical serotonin within the brain. Additional research indicates that other soil-based microorganisms—such as *Mycobacterium vaccae*—can improve quality of life, depression, and anxiety when orally consumed by adult cancer patients.

Although a wide variety of microorganisms, including *Lactobacillus* and *Bifidobacteria,* are found in soil, our fear of contamination can make us unwilling to touch soil. This may be limiting our exposure to them, in yet another form of modern nature deprivation. International scientists have concluded that our antibacterial world is contributing to the massive rise in allergies and that lack of exposure to microbes can alter normal immune system balance. Much more research is required, but it is becoming increasingly clear that incidental and purposeful contact with soil through gardening activities—digging in it, breathing it in, letting it touch our skin—provides a portal for beneficial bacteria to gain access to the nasal passages and gastrointestinal tract, a gardening reality that may have far-reaching consequences for the human brain. We are long past the time when the difference between soil and dirt should be a point of confusion: soil must no longer be confused with dirt. It is a living, breathing form of nature.

## Gardening and Cognition

Enhanced cognitive functioning is yet another benefit gardening activities provide. Gardening presents cognitive challenges requiring memorization, visuospatial skills, and executive functioning. Using these cognitive attributes helps to place a layer of protection against the forces of brain aging. In a study published in the *Journal of the American Geriatrics Society* in 1995, gardening was associated with a 50 percent reduction in dementia risk among older adults. Even among patients with known Alzheimer's disease, participation in a horticultural therapy program (twice weekly for three months) has been shown to improve cognitive functioning compared with controls. Because dementia can compromise cognitive abilities required for gardening, supervision and proper instruction by a qualified horticultural therapist is a key component to care.

---

### Dr. Eva's File

Martha, my 70-year-old patient, said, "There is nothing like working the earth with my hands and knowing that I will eventually be enjoying those beautiful red tomatoes. When I am in my garden, it feels like time doesn't exist."

---

At the other end of life's spectrum—in childhood—gardening is equally valuable for cognitive functioning. A century ago, gardening programs blossomed in North American schools. The gardens were not a recess playground or set up for mere leisure; they were incorporated as an educational tool. As stated by one of the school gardening pioneers, Herbert Hemenway, in 1906: "It not only educates the head, the heart and the hand, but it aids in practical application of reading, writing and arithmetic. Gardening increases and develops the power of observation. It makes a person quick to grasp ideas and put these ideas into action. Boys and girls having gardens have been found to be more rapid in mental, physical and moral development . . . it opens up a source of revenue, creates a love of industry, and respect for property, and is often the beginning of better things."

Hartford, Connecticut school administrator Hemenway was not alone in his beliefs. Toward the end of World War I, school gardens and summer garden educational programs were thriving across North America. The boom was driven by President Woodrow Wilson's directive establishing a national School Garden Army. Some 4 million boys and girls signed up to work under its motto "A Garden for Every Child—Every Child in a Garden." Although its original primary directive was to produce food during wartime, it soon became clear to its operator, the U.S. Bureau of Education, that the program had immense educational value. More than a year after World War I ended, while the program scraped by on a bare budget, the School Garden Army director, John L. Randall, made the case for permanency, stating that "gardening admits the widest kind of correlation with other studies. There is no school subject from which more real knowledge can be gained of science, of art, of life's relations than of dealing with living, growing plants." However, the program was disbanded in 1921 when government money dried up.

In 1948, Harold B. Tukey, the president of the American Society for Horticultural Science and a highly respected scientist, expressed concern that the art of horticulture and it social and educational values were being cast aside in the boom of technology, stating that it "is being pushed aside by too many. We become so involved in the biological and affairs side that we overlook the one that is likely to be the most important in the years immediately ahead . . . gardening means health, stability, and happiness." Tukey contended that horticulture allows broad connectivity in learning and human growth because it removes isolation in scientific education. Connecting with the environment through gardening allows students to see the broad implications and meaning of their studies, leading to a better understanding of different scientific subjects.

Until the late 1960s, there was little scientific proof to support the contention that school gardens enhance cognitive and academic achievement. In 1968, researchers in Dearborn, Michigan, administered a 55-question knowledge test to almost 300 public school students who had been enrolled in one of three groups: hands-on school gardening, classroom-only gardening instruction, or no access to either hands-on or classroom gardening instruction. The results of the investigation showed that hands-on gardening produced far better retention and assimilation of facts and skills related to the principles and practice of gardening than did classroom-only instruction.

It would take several decades before school gardening would be the subject of more focused research. The results would be worth the wait. In separate studies published in 2005 in *HortTechnology,* both a 14-week school gardening program and a single academic-year gardening program elevated overall science achievement scores among elementary students, thus confirming the scientific liaison effect proposed by Tukey. In addition to improved scores on standardized science testing, contemporary research also shows brain-boosting effects of school gardens in factors that encourage broad problem solving. In the real world—academic and employment settings in particular—the ability to understand one's actions and appreciate their implications and the ability to work in groups are key attributes to successful problem solving, to seeing things from another angle, and to communicating effectively. Although high test scores are academically desirable, the broader challenge in the real world is to apply, communicate, and collaborate with that knowledge. A single academic-year gardening program has been shown to enhance overall life skills, the ability to work in groups, and self-understanding when compared with a control group of elementary schoolchildren without hands-on gardening education.

## Gardening Changes the Brain for Life

There are long-term consequences to a brain shaped by gardening experience in youth—it changes how children eat and how they think about the planet. In examining a single academic-year gardening program (the 1996–97 school year), researchers at Texas A&M University found that elementary students who had experience with seeds, planting and transplanting, using garden tools, and caring for plants in raised garden beds displayed more positive environmental attitudes than school students who were not exposed to the garden intervention. These results take on greater meaning when placed in the context of a study published in 2005 in *HortTechnology*, which involved randomly selected adults living in metropolitan areas (average age 42). Those adults who reported having participated in active gardening as children were more likely to consider trees to have mental health and personal value, and they were more likely to engage in gardening as adults. Moreover, when elementary school students had more frequent educational sessions at local farms during an academic year, they subsequently had more positive attitudes concerning locally grown produce and an affinity toward the regions where farms are located. Any experience that improves the attitudes of children toward local foods and the natural environments in which they are grown can only be a good thing, and the beneficial environmental and economic implications may be untold.

Add to this the multiple studies showing that gardening influences dietary habits, and in particular the willingness to eat fruits and vegetables. In the last five years, the results of various studies have been incredibly consistent: children who are involved in gardening programs at school and beyond subsequently have improved recognition and knowledge of, as well as preferences for, healthy vegetables. Indeed, increased vegetable consumption in gardeners appears to extend to older adults (50 years or older) as well. There are, of course, multiple health benefits to a greater consumption of healthy produce, which we focus on in the next chapter.

## Wilderness and Adventure Therapy

Gardening may be considered a tame form of nature contact, and at the other end of the continuum sits the equally beneficial encounters with nature in the wild form. The origins of contemporary wilderness and adventure therapy in North America take us back to the wilderness prescriptions of famed medical doctor and author S. Weir Mitchell. His article "Camp Cure" was published in *Lippincott's* magazine in 1874 and ultimately became a popular book under the same title. Weir contended that due to wear and tear on the nervous system, many overworked city dwellers needed more than a visit to a local park or a day trip to the countryside. He referred to these efforts as an incomplete or weak form of nature remedy, one that would suffice for some but not match the needs of many emotionally and cognitively taxed urbanites. Rather, a more complete prescription was one akin to pressing a mental reset button, brought on by "a healthful change for a time in the mode of living." The time generally involved a couple of weeks, and the mode of living change involved giving up four walls for a tent.

Weir's camp cure wasn't a matter of packing up and heading off into the wilderness on an unprepared, ill-advised solo effort. It was to be conducted with experienced guides. Within it there would be opportunity for solitude and reflection, as well as social connectivity with others in camp. Weir suggested that the benefits could be magnified by keeping a mindful mental record of the sights, sounds, and scents encountered. He advised anyone involved in the camp cure "to keep a diary not of events, but of things," citing, for example, "that the sun against the sloped yellow bank has covered the water with a shining changeful orange light, through which shine the mottled stones below, and that the concave curve of every wave that faces us concentrates for the eye an unearthly sapphire the reflex of the darkening blue above us." Weir was prescribing mindfulness in the wilderness.

The camp cure—or wilderness cure, as it would come to be known—maintained its popularity and continued to be referenced in medical textbooks as a potential therapy for depressive symptoms. However, in the early 1900s, camp therapy for many urbanites gave way to sanitariums, which offered a slightly more comfortable way to tap into the therapeutic aspects of nature during extended stays.

Also in the early part of the 20th century, U.S. state and local corrections officials initiated forest camp programs for juvenile delinquents and low-risk adult offenders. In 1935, California became the first state to legislate a formal forest camp program for youth offenders. By 1960, forest camp programs for rehabilitation were thriving in over a dozen states. (With time and experience, authorities were able to screen individuals to determine which were most likely to succeed in such minimum-security environments.) Administrators reported their forest camp programs to be successful on many levels; these efforts included conservation activities that provided participants with a sense of purpose and meaning, enhanced their ability to work with others, and improved resourcefulness and self-confidence. At least anecdotally it became clear that the outdoor experience acted as a preventive measure in keeping at-risk youth on the right side of the law.

In the early 1960s, Outward Bound and other groups began challenge-based educational and skills-building programs in natural settings for members of the general public. Soon, wilderness therapy was once again being discussed in psychiatric circles as a means of promoting mental health. In 1967, psychiatrist Robert C. Martin from Stockton State Hospital for mental health in California set out with 10 colleagues and 74 patients for the forests of Lake Alpine in the Sierra Nevada. Martin and his colleagues wrote about their experiences and the positive changes in patient mood, motivation, social interaction, and behavior. They also reported a profound observation about mental-health-care providers: "Of all the benefits derived from the camping trip," Martin stated, "the most lasting and significant appears to be the changed perception of patients by staff . . . The staff, too, behaved differently outside the confines of the hospital role. They were more likely to interact like people with people, instead of like staff with patients. That, perhaps, was the greatest advantage of the experience." Martin's observation gets at the heart and soul of the burgeoning ecotherapy (ecopsychiatry, ecopsychology) movement, which stresses the importance of conducting individual and group psychotherapy sessions in nature or greenspace settings. (We discuss ecotherapy in further detail in Chapter 9.)

In 1975, Outward Bound modified some of its programs to suit the needs of mental health patients, and many were subsequently attached by physicians to clinical programs in major hospitals and community mental health programs. The Outward Bound Mental Health Project involved taking great care to, at least objectively, select patients best suited to such excursions, and trips typically lasted a few days, rather than the two to four weeks of standard Outward Bound programs. Favorable results continued to be published in various medical and psychological journals, and the general understanding was that wilderness-adventure challenge was a form of adjunctive medicine—it was not the primary treatment; rather, it was one that could enhance the likelihood of clinical success. Commenting on their successful four-day program, a group of psychologists from New York's Rockland County Community Mental Health Center stated in 1984, "The Wilderness Challenge was designed to mesh with the preexisting treatment plan . . . it is easy to let such a wilderness-based experience degenerate into purely recreational activity. Careful planning and staffing prior to the outing and constant vigilance and staff communication during it are necessary to ensure maximum therapeutic benefit as well as an enjoyable and safe adventure."

Wilderness experience as a defined therapy is serious business, and there was detailed work to be done to ensure its success. Despite the challenges, wilderness-adventure interventions as a form of adjunctive medicine in mental health care enjoy an impressive adherence record—among patients with serious forms of mental illness, the treatment adherence tops 97 percent and dropouts are rare. Nature-based interventions aren't akin to pharmaceutical drugs, but one would be hard-pressed to find any mainstream psychotherapeutic intervention, drugs or otherwise, with compliance rates over 90 percent.

### Dr. Eva's File

Adam was 17 years old. His mother was concerned about his drug use and that he was failing school. She had tried sending him to a therapist, but it seemed he was beyond help. She was at her wit's end, having just gotten through an ugly three-year divorce battle. Adam's father was of little help, as he had addiction issues himself. She feared Adam was one step from being caught by the law and possibly incarcerated. I suggested that she look into wilderness programs for youths, where he could learn respect for nature and for himself. In such a program, Adam would need to learn how to survive and to listen—and most of all, he could gain self-esteem and appreciation for others and for the world he lives in.

That summer, Adam very reluctantly went to wilderness camp. Not surprisingly, he returned a different person—a man. Responsible and wanting to go back to school. Wanting to make a difference.

# A Higher Dose of Forest Medicine

*For the millions who labor in the store and factory*
*and office we must provide recreation grounds where*
*these toilers can find a relaxation from the fearful*
*nervous and mental strain that is their lot, and so*
*we turn to the calm and inspiration of our natural*
*forest, the antithesis of our modern city life, and seek*
*again the inspiration and recreation that was once*
*the privilege of every American to seek and find.*
—Ottomar Van Norden, *Journal of the New York State*
*Forestry Association,* 1916

Typically, the studies involving the physiological and psychological changes induced by shinrin-yoku—contemplation and/or physical activity in the forest—have involved time frames of only a few hours or half a day. For the camp cure physician, S. Weir Mitchell, an hour or so in an urban park might be considered "the remedy in weak form." In recent years, Korean researchers have been investigating the effects of a higher dose of what is now referred to as forest medicine (most of the veteran shinrin-yoku researchers have adopted the name; see www.infom.org).

Won Sop Shin, a graduate of the University of Toronto forestry PhD program, is now one of the leading experts in forest medicine. In a series of studies, Dr. Shin and colleagues from Korea found that five-day forest camping programs (some with challenges such as rock climbing and hiking, as well as group activities) have proven effective in improving depression among otherwise healthy college students and in adults with alcohol addiction. Working with physicians, they have established a nine-day forest program that begins with simple forest experience in the camp. Days three to six offer adventure challenges, and for the wind down, from days seven to nine, there is an introspection component involving meditation and counseling within the forest setting. In controlled research published in 2011 in *Environmental Health and Preventive Medicine,* the reduction in depression scores after the nine-day forest intervention was a very meaningful 64 percent. Consider that a 50 percent or more reduction in depression scores is considered the gold standard in drug trials. This combination of systematic nature-based recreation, challenge, and psychotherapy may be the intervention of the future, an updated and refined version of the camp cure.

## What Makes Wilderness Effective?

We are obviously proponents of nature and nature-based medical interventions, but we're also the first to admit that it would be easy to pick apart the methodological flaws of the wilderness-adventure studies. Within the scientific literature there are nearly as many publications criticizing the lack of iron-clad research design in wilderness-adventure studies as there are actual wilderness intervention studies. We are hopeful that scientists will continue to use creative research designs to allow for greater inspection of the true value of wilderness experiences. The solution, however, is not simple: wilderness-adventure therapy is not a drug with a simple chemical structure that can be compared with a sugar pill in those with depression. It becomes very difficult to secure a proper control group for interventions that involve such a wide variety of variables that might also account for post-wilderness success. Evidentiary debates aside, there seems little dispute that wilderness experience can stimulate positive emotions and is an opportunity to bring the mind from internal symptoms, suffering of the past, and anxiety of the future. Wilderness provides an environment well suited to mindfulness and bite-size spans of keeping the mind in the present moment. Theoretically, even if the joy reported by patients is only transitory, just a few fleeting moments, it may be just enough to allow for another mental vantage point. It can let depressed individuals know that joy is possible, that it's something within reach.

Although much more research is required before the scientific community can determine the ways in which forest medicine and wilderness-adventure therapies work to promote mental health, the emerging research shows that their value is an extension of their ability to restore and rejuvenate the brain. Dr. Stephen Kaplan's attention restoration theory states that natural environments are restorative by virtue of several factors: being away from the usual environment (unless your wilderness adventure is just down the street, this should be easily fulfilled), provocation of fascination, extent or vastness of the natural environment, and its ability to fulfill the purpose and expectations of individuals. In particular, the positive psychology benefits can be maximized when the natural environment provokes fascination and deeply engages the mind. The more closely a wilderness-adventure therapy environment meets Kaplan's attention restoration theory criteria, the better the results might be.

As important as the group dynamic may be within wilderness programs, it also seems reasonable to suspect that opportunity for individual solitude, reflection, and contemplation are critical features. In the U.S. Wilderness Act of 1964, Congress specifically mandated that wilderness areas be designated, among other reasons, to "provide opportunities for solitude, and to provide a primitive and unconfined type of recreation." Solitude has been unfairly tarnished in modern times, often associated with loneliness and social isolation, and ultimately something to be feared. In our gadget-driven world, where we often feel we must stay connected and informed, solitude becomes uncomfortable—we're culturally groomed to avoid it. Solitude amid wilderness is just what the doctor *should* order, however. Research indicates that solitude in the wilderness—the personal choice to experience some solitude in a natural setting—provides a later insulation from the social structures and environments that can overwhelm us. Solitude is, of course, best served up in small doses. The editors of an 1865 issue of *Current Literature* captured it best under the title "The Service of Solitude—Regeneration through Reflection": "If solitude be looked upon from a wholesome point of view, it will be seen that it is of real value only as a tonic. We do not take quinine with the intention of living for the rest of our born days as the slave of that drug, and no man should retire to a cave with the purpose of making it his residence."

Undoubtedly, the benefits of wilderness-adventure interventions can be ascribed to many of the nature factors discussed to this point in this book. Experiencing the aesthetically pleasing sights, natural sounds (or absence of noise), aromatic scents, invisible negative ions, natural light and darkness, animals, and so on can all elevate the benefits of physical activity and resiliency-building challenges inherent in such programs.

---

### A Note of Caution

A critical factor in wilderness adventure as a successful form of nature therapy is the human operational factor. There is a massive difference between a wilderness-adventure camp run by well-intentioned, outdoor-enthusiast entrepreneurs and one that is structured and staffed by highly trained professionals. The broad divide between these extremes remains murky—and potentially fatal. The potential rejuvenating influences of nature can be quickly undone by a mismatch between a client and a charlatan hiding behind the veil of marketing images. Even S. Weir Mitchell called for professional guides in his prescriptions. But almost a century and a half later, there remains little regulation over these programs, and colorful, impressive brochures, websites, and slogans do not equate to a successful and safe wilderness-adventure program. Less than half of North American states and provinces license wilderness guides and outfitters. Even where licensing does exist, its validity may be dubious, since only a few jurisdictions require even first-aid training as a condition of licensure. Regardless of the intent when signing up for a wilderness-adventure experience, be it for mental rejuvenation or adjunctive care of a mental health issue, clients must beware: move past the glossy pictures of brochures and websites and have a look at the training, experience, and qualifications of the operators.

---

# Gardening and Wilderness—Self, Community, Planet

Gardening or experiencing time in the wilderness offers benefits to the self, the community, and ultimately, the planet. These activities promote self-awareness, positive mood, and creativity; diminish stress; and improve cognition. A cognitively restored and refreshed brain is primed for empathy; one that is drained, overwhelmed, and multitasking is empathically disarmed. When conducted in groups, these activities create a bond and sense of community among participants. Groups working together in gardens beautify communities and strengthen bonds, while wilderness-adventure group experiences also teach the importance of self-sacrifice and community strength. Indeed, development of sense of community is a predictor of overall satisfaction with wilderness-adventure experiences. All of this feeds forward a change, or at the very least, a reinforcement of environmental knowledge and pro-environmental attitudes. Outdoor programs, gardening, and wilderness encourage empathy for the planet.

8

# The Brain on Nature's Nutrients:
# Nutri-Ecopsychology

*The ancient Athenian grew wise and strong in
intellect so long as he partook simply of the plain diet
afforded from the Mediterranean Sea, his
own hills of Greece, and from the pleasant pastures of
his native land . . . the Esquimau eats the fat of the
seal and walrus, and maintains a serene mental
front . . . the inhabitants of the sunny South subsist
on the orange, the bread-fruit, the banana and fish
from river and sea; and we find in them but slight
development of mental disorders.*
—Selden H. Talcott, MD, New York, 1888

For over a century, North American physicians have made note
of the various ways in which nutrition may influence cognition and
brain fatigue, improve short-term mental outlook, and protect against
long-term depression and anxiety. In particular, early researchers were
intrigued by the most appropriate diet for offsetting mentally taxing
office work. By the end of the 1800s, fish was the most consistently
cited brain food. In his famous 1873 book *Foods,* highly regarded
British physician Edward Smith stated that "the value of fish as a

part of the dietary is... especially fitted for those who perform much brain work, or who are the victims of much anxiety and distress." Writing in 1897 in the *Woman's Medical Journal,* physicians promoted apples, prunes, tomatoes, almonds, and walnuts as primary foods for cognitive function and support of the brain and nervous system. Commercial interests became involved in the promotion of whole grains for mental performance; for example, Grape-Nuts cereal was heavily marketed in magazines as a "food for brain and nerve centers." Collectively, they were essentially promoting the key aspects of what we now call the Mediterranean diet: whole grains, fish and other seafood, seeds and nuts, and colorful fruits and vegetables.

A century before our modern-day battles on the open plains of the Internet—the verbal sword swinging between those ascribing to veganism and their adversaries, the meat-hungry proponents of the Paleolithic diet—experts disagreed over the ultimate brain diet. Lady Paget Walburga, a close friend of England's Queen Victoria, advocated for the clear thinking provided by a strictly plant-based diet, cautioning that a meat diet "trammels and materializes our higher faculties." Others saw it differently, suggesting that animal meat was a necessity for optimal mental performance. The 1871 editors of *Scientific American* provided some fish-friendly middle ground, stating that "it is well known that certain kinds of foods are peculiarly fitted for keeping the brain in a state of healthy activity... fish, fruit, vegetables, milk, and the various kinds of farinaceous foods, graham bread and oatmeal taking the lead. Some constitutions, however, seem to thrive on a strictly vegetable diet." All were in agreement, however, that the diet should be as close to nature (i.e., unprocessed) as possible, not taken in excess quantities, and devoid of the processed sweets that were becoming increasingly common.

Leonard Hill, a leading physician of the early 1900s, was concerned that nature deprivation and physical inactivity among urban office workers was being compounded "by indulgence in food, e.g., sweets which are everywhere to his hand." Hill and a handful of other physicians and scientists sensed a shift, one that would be proven in our own time: as countries develop and rural residents migrate to urban centers, the transition is accompanied by the need for convenience, leading to an increase in consumption of processed foods, sugar, animal fat, and lower-nutrient meals that are prepared away from the home. As fountain-shop delicacies and soft drinks entered mainstream diets, some in the medical community were waving a red flag about the consequences of a shift toward sugar, processed foods, and food additives. The physician editors of *Medical Standard* in 1922 took a particularly hard line, that what is not for us is against us:

> *In matters of so vital import as diet, nothing should be taken for granted... every time we allow our children or ourselves to indulge in the output of the candy shop, soda fountain or pastry counter, we introduce into their lives those very elements that corrupt and undermine their existence... indulgence in denatured, devitalized and demoralized foodstuffs. In other words, any kind of food is unfit to eat when its composition, through some artificial form of kitchen treatment, has become hostile to physiological life and incompatible to enter into the creative processes of human nature. For food which is not creative is destructive... the field which at present, more than any other, offers the individual an opportunity to gain or lose, rise or fall in his dealing with destiny, is the field of diet.*

The editors of *Medical Standard* could obviously sense a change at play, yet even they couldn't have dreamed where we were heading and the extent to which denatured and devitalized food and drink would surround us in our contemporary technological world.

## It's All Part of a Balanced Diet

The notion of brain foods, at least in their whole-food form, fell out of favor in the mid-20th century, cast out into a pseudoscientific purgatory until the 1980s. Outside of concerns over overt deficiencies of vitamins and minerals, few physicians and scientists took seriously the lingering ideas of food as a mediator of cognitive and mental health. In fact, scientists presented isolated stimulants, highly processed carbohydrates, soft drinks, candy and other products of technological processing to the North American public as the *answer* to brain fatigue. Consider the 1944 magazine headline "Vendors dispense brain food: Candy and soft drinks get scientific rating by AAAS." The AAAS is the American Association for the Advancement of Science, and some of its scientists concluded at their annual meeting that "a sugar meal, frequently taken in the form of a soft drink or candy, will maintain cerebral efficiency." As long as a food or beverage was capable of getting sugar up into the brain, it could be considered a brain food.

American druggists, some of whom were now also in the business of running soda shops, presented science indicating that carbonated soft drinks had antimicrobial properties. They presumed such beverages could bolster immunity and prevent depressive symptoms common to those feeling run-down. Media added to the hype, with headlines such as "Soda fountain optimism" and "Benefits of the soda fountain"—in soda, they told us, was resiliency against depression. Who needed fish, apples, almonds, and whole grains when candy and stimulants could fuel the brain?

There were, of course, still foods considered to be healthy, and they were juxtaposed against an ever-expanding list of nonnutritious foods and drinks. This bloated list of items, all increasingly separated from nature, could be consumed as part of the proverbial "balanced diet." Gone was the idea that in the dietary realm what was not for us was against us. Viewed under favorable marketing light, junk food was something that energized the brain, and dietetic groups dismissed the worst of it as completely benign, as long as it was consumed along with equal parts of "something healthy." Never mind that individuals adhering to a balanced diet were becoming as elusive as the Sasquatch. Scientists also told us not to worry about the dyes, chemical preservatives, and artificial ingredients in our processed food; any purported reaction was surely a figment of the imagination.

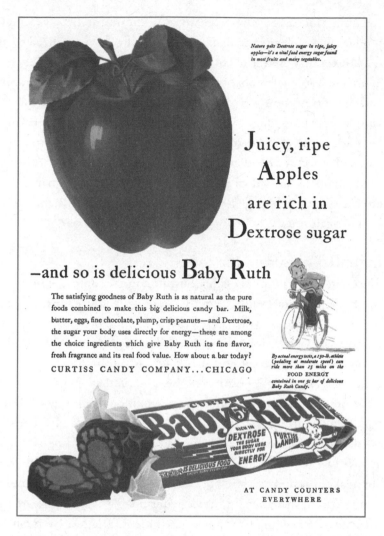

Nature puts Dextrose sugar in ripe, juicy apples—it's a vital food energy sugar found in most fruits and many vegetables.

Juicy, ripe Apples are rich in Dextrose sugar

—and so is delicious Baby Ruth

The satisfying goodness of Baby Ruth is as natural as the pure foods combined to make this big delicious candy bar. Milk, butter, eggs, fine chocolate, plump, crisp peanuts—and Dextrose, the sugar your body uses directly for energy—these are among the choice ingredients which give Baby Ruth its fine flavor, fresh fragrance and its real food value. How about a bar today?

CURTISS CANDY COMPANY...CHICAGO

By actual energy tests, a 150-lb. athlete (pedaling at moderate speed) can ride more than 15 miles on the FOOD ENERGY contained in one 5c bar of delicious Baby Ruth Candy.

AT CANDY COUNTERS
EVERYWHERE

The shift from whole foods to a place where a candy bar became akin to an apple (see the Baby Ruth advertisement from 1940) was the dawning of a new era, another form of nature deprivation with consequences that we are only just now starting to come to grips with. We have turned our backs on the nutrition of nature, that which helped us thrive during our evolution. As we process away nature in all its forms, including the dietary, we pay a physical price in the form of low-grade inflammation. This smoldering inflammation, as it is referred to by some researchers, is a by-product of the changes to diet and lifestyle that have occurred over the last century, and it is not without brain-health consequences. There are also environmental consequences to our dietary habits and the agribusiness we currently support. We discuss this below and also provide a message of hope: If we can reconnect with nature by returning to whole foods, with a lean toward the Mediterranean diet and aspects of the diet consumed by our Paleolithic ancestors, the benefits to individual and planetary health will be many. We are past the time of urgency for a return to the foods that are for us, not against us.

## Essential Natural Nutrients

The brain implications of quality nutrition in the context of positive psychology, mental health, cognition, ecology, and sustainability are now scientifically convincing, yet they remain underappreciated by many. Massive transformations in the last 50 years have obviously changed the way we eat and drink—there are both excesses and deficiencies in the composition of the modern diet. We are still far removed from the consumption of the traditional brain foods: fish, whole grains, fruits, vegetables, nuts, and seeds. Certainly, there is no shortage of choice when it comes to merely providing calories as raw fuel to the brain—if it were only so simple. Despite the abundance of choice technology has provided us, despite swimming in a sea of inexpensive and rapidly consumable calories, we are in many ways drowning from malnourishment. The relative malnutrition presents itself as a void in the areas of essential fats, fiber, and anti-inflammatory and antioxidant phytonutrients from fruits, vegetables, and nuts.

### Essential Fats

Omega-3 and omega-6 fatty acids are essential for human health and brain functioning. These groups are known as essential fats because we cannot produce them on our own and so must be obtained through dietary intake. Omega-3 fatty acids are found in relative abundance in fish, seafood, free-range eggs, wild game and open-pasture meat, flaxseed, walnuts, chia seeds, purslane, and to some degree in various other berries, nuts, and seeds. Linoleic acid, the primary omega-6 fatty acid, is found in abundance in safflower, sunflower, soybean, and corn oils. In our hunter-gatherer past, we had an omega-6 to omega-3 intake ratio that was fairly close to 1:1. It was an intake that facilitated development and optimal functioning in the human brain and, based on anthropological records, one that we have maintained fairly consistently until recent decades. However, the introduction of cheap, highly processed omega-6 vegetable oils and changes in animal-rearing practices have skewed this evolutionary ratio. Today, the omega-6 to omega-3 ratio is at least 10 parts, and up to 20 parts, omega-6 for every one part omega-3. It is an unacceptable ratio, one far removed from the ideal ratio near 1:1 recommended in 1999 by an international panel of lipid experts in the *Journal of the American College of Nutrition.*

The high omega-6 ratio is fueled by the reality that our vegetable oil intake has tripled since the early 1960s. We now consume 48 1/2 pounds of soybean oil annually per person—versus 13 pounds per year just 50 years ago. On the other hand, the average intake of the two key omega-3 fatty acids—eicosapentaenoic and docosahexaenoic acids (EPAs and DHAs respectively)—in North America is only 130 milligrams per day. This level is more than 500 milligrams short of the guidelines set by the aforementioned panel of experts, and over 800 milligrams short of the 1,000 milligrams recommended by the American Heart Association for those with heart disease. Highly processed vegetable oils surround us in baked goods, fried foods, snacks, and salad dressings—if oil is added to food somewhere along the line, chances are good that it is a linoleic acid–rich omega-6 oil. Animals, including fish, that are allowed to graze, hunt and peck, forage, or swim uninhibited have access to the naturally occurring omega-3 fatty acids in grasses, insects, algae, and other natural sources, but the meats and eggs from confined animals and farmed fish have much higher levels of omega-6 than they normally would, thanks to grain-feeding practices. Unless you are a vegan, you are what you eat eats.

Countless international studies have shown that as important as omega-6 fatty acids are, once a line is crossed into excess, they can influence the production of inflammatory chemicals. Even the low-grade production of inflammatory immune chemicals (cytokines) can compromise a healthy mental outlook. Depression and anxiety are characterized by an overproduction of inflammatory chemicals. Excess omega-6 fatty acids, particularly in the relative absence of omega-3 fatty acids, therefore have the potential to play a role in a number of neurological and psychiatric conditions. Omega-3 fatty acids, on the other hand, have been shown to have an anti-inflammatory impact in the body and to be beneficial in a number of behavioral and neurological conditions. Because dietary fats influence the structure and functioning of brain cells, this preponderance of omega-6 and relative deficiency of omega-3 has, as we discuss below, consequences in the realm of mental and cognitive health.

## Whole Grains and Sugar

> *It is well known that too much sugar causes tooth decay, but might it also cause "brain decay"? Recent research suggests that it just might.*
> —Janet Jankowiak, MD, editorial in *Neurology,* 2004

Much is made these days about whether a product contains "whole grain," and with good reason. Fiber-rich whole grains are associated with lower inflammatory chemicals in the body. Whole grains are also a potent source of antioxidant chemicals. The connection between a diet rich in whole grains and a decreased risk of diabetes, cardiovascular disease, and obesity has been well documented. Since the Made with Whole Grains! logo adorns just about everything these days, including high-sugar cereals that may or may not have a cartoon character on the package, one would presume that we are indulging heavily on the whole-grain front. Sadly, it isn't true. Although we obtain a good portion of our daily caloric intake in the form of cereal grains—they account for about a quarter of our total percentage energy intake—only a miniscule 3.5 percent of our energy from grains is consumed in the form of whole grains. That means 96.5 percent of our grain intake is in the form of processed grains.

## Percentage of Nutrients in Whole Wheat Flour and White Flour

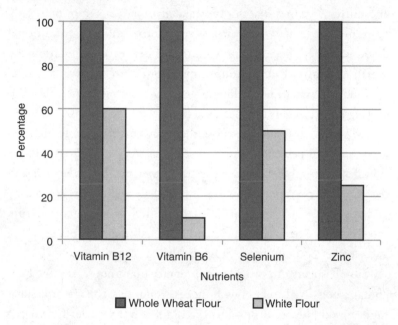

When flour is processed, nature's brain-supportive nutrients (B vitamins, selenium, zinc) and fiber are torn off. (Inadequate levels of any one of these nutrients has been associated with depression.) Then, in a sort of nutritional shell game, some manufacturers throw a touch of whole grain back into their processed breads, snacks, and cereals, among other foods, so they can claim "Whole grains!" on the packaging. When this buzzword is emblazoned on a package, it certainly implies that the contents are part of a balanced diet. The consumer perceives that the product is a healthy, fiber-rich, low-sugar grain product. Unfortunately, these logos are nutritionally meaningless. Consider candy-like cereals—a dusting of whole-grain flour "justifies" the manufacturer-styled Whole Grains stamp, and the visual disguises the reality that a small serving contains 15-plus grams of sugar and only a single gram of fiber. According to the U.S. Food and Drug Administration (FDA), a product can be called whole grain if it is 51 percent whole grain by weight. This is not to be confused with "contains whole grain," which could mean as little as a few molecules to a few milligrams. When we see past the smoke and mirrors, we find that our typical daily fiber consumption is only 13 grams—at least 33 percent less than those following traditional diets consumed a century ago. Current fiber recommendations by North American dietetic groups range from 21 to 38 grams per day.

One thing we are not lacking is sugar. Our overall intake of insulin-spiking refined sugars has increased by eightfold in the last 200 years. Added sugars, distinct from those that occur naturally in foods, now account for 16 percent of our daily calories. As a reference point for this absurd number, consider that the American Heart Association recommends no more than 5 percent of daily energy be supplied by added sugars. Our per annum intake of high-fructose corn syrup, often added to beverages, increased from half a pound per capita in 1970 to over 60 pounds per capita by the late 1990s.

Simple sugars can provide a temporary brain boost, but the benefits are short-lived and not without consequence. Soon after the sugar high, blood glucose drops and the brain is left wondering what is going on—empty calories become an empty promise that cannot be sustained. On the other hand, fiber-rich whole grains break down slowly, do not spike blood insulin levels, and provide a more consistent supply of energy and vital nutrients. With constant sugary spikes in insulin, our cells can become less responsive to the hormone and even higher levels of insulin are needed to guide sugar into our cells. Making a habit out of stringing together quick sugar fixes as brain food can catch up with us in an insulin resistance triad: cardiovascular disease, diabetes, and abdominal obesity. Lack of fiber and consistently elevated blood insulin is associated with inflammation and risk of cognitive decline and depression.

## Colorful Fruits, Vegetables, and Phytochemicals

The fruit and vegetable story is even sadder than the whole-grain and essential fat debacle. Four dietary items account for half of the total vegetable intake among U.S. adults: potatoes (mostly frozen and fried), iceberg lettuce, onions, and tomatoes. Despite the efforts of government and private nutrition education groups to encourage us to increase our intake of fruits and vegetables, we continue to bypass colorful produce. Eliminating potatoes from the equation, only 29 percent of adults and 13 percent of children consume 5 servings of any other fruits and vegetables per day. Because we aren't meeting the general 7 to 10 servings guideline on fruit and vegetable intake, it should be no surprise that we are oceans away from meeting the gold standard U.S. Department of Agriculture recommendations of consuming five major dietary colors groups (reds, greens, orange/yellows, purple/blues, non-potato whites) per day.

Nutritional scientists and educators advocate for a variety of colorful plant foods because they contain naturally occurring chemicals called phytochemicals. In unprocessed whole foods, these microchemicals give plants their color, taste, and texture and provide us with vital antioxidant and anti-inflammatory support. You can see these chemicals as the deep red and purple colors of fresh grapes, blueberries, cherries, and beets; the deep green in spinach and kale; the orange in carrots and squash; the whites in radishes and roots; and the yellow in corn. We can fully tap into the health-promoting properties of these chemicals only by consuming a range of colorful plants. Unfortunately, the most comprehensive study of its kind, published in 2006 in the *Journal of the American Dietetic Association*, showed that the average combined daily servings of dark green and deeply colored orange and yellow vegetables is only a meager one and a half servings. And in a study published in the *Journal of Cancer*

*Education* in 2007 involving over 1,600 parents, not a single one consumed the five major dietary color groups most days of the week (i.e., more than three and a half days per week), and only 40 percent of parents and 26 percent of children ate from the five major color groups over the course of an entire week.

## For Us or Against Us—Changing the Brain with Foods

> *It is both compelling and daunting to consider that dietary intervention at an individual or population level could reduce rates of psychiatric disorders. There are exciting implications for clinical care, public health, and research.*
>
> —Marlene P. Freeman, MD, Harvard Medical School, editorial in *American Journal of Psychiatry,* 2010

Scientists continue to map out the complex mechanisms through which foods can work for or against our brain cells. At the heart of this work is the ability of foods and beverages to either promote or prevent oxidative stress and inflammation. As we have previously discussed, when inflammatory chemicals are elevated at even low levels in otherwise healthy, well-adjusted adults, depressive symptoms, anxiety, and brain fog are often the end result. Mental health disorders and cognitive decline are associated with ongoing low-grade inflammation, or as researchers call it, neuro-inflammation. Oxidative stress is also emerging as a common thread among various neurological and emotional disorders. Free radical production (oxidative stress) is a consequence of oxygen use in normal day-to-day living and breathing, and is normally kept in check by elaborate antioxidant pathways in the body. The lack of sufficient antioxidants can cause oxidative stress to alter the structure and function of delicate nerve cells.

Inflammation and oxidative stress are not mutually exclusive. They represent a vicious cycle: oxidative stress promotes inflammation and vice versa. The constant stress of low-grade inflammation and oxidative stress overburdens the brain's protection and repair systems. For example, brain-derived neurotrophic factor (BDNF), the nerve growth factor that supports the growth and survival of our nerve cells, is diminished by neuro-inflammation. Eventually, the oxidative stress-inflammation cycle causes small but meaningful changes to the nerve cell structure. Oxidative stress also appears to accelerate the breakdown of mood-regulating neurotransmitters such as serotonin and dopamine.

To summarize, inflammation and oxidative stress can influence the brain in two main ways: by changing the structure of brain cells and by changing the availability of the chemicals that bind to those nerve cells and facilitate nerve cell communication. Structural changes affect the way the neurotransmitters "fit" into the receptors on the nerve cells—think of the neurotransmitter like a key going into a lock. If the key does not fit the lock smoothly, proper nerve-to-nerve communication may be slightly compromised and this may manifest as mood or behavioral change. Lowered availability of neurotransmitters can also negatively influence mood and cognition.

Scientists are developing drugs for mental health and various forms of dementia based on their ability to stem neuro-inflammation. Antidepressant and antianxiety medications may curb neuro-inflammation because they offer antioxidant and anti-inflammatory properties. Yet, there are underappreciated dietary ways to support the structure and functioning of nerve cells. Phytochemicals, abundant in the colorful fruits and vegetables many of us shun, are strong antioxidant and anti-inflammatory agents and have recently been shown to turn down the fires of neuro-inflammation and prevent the rapid breakdown of our mood-regulating brain chemicals. Omega-3 fats, fiber-rich grains, roots, and legumes can also effectively turn down the dial on neuro-inflammation. Components within the foods that work for us influence the way mood-regulating neurotransmitters work and the extent to which they remain active. Because inflammation and oxidative stress can be controlled to a meaningful extent by diet and the entire workings of the antioxidant defense system is controlled by dietary nutrients, we can change our brains for the better by keeping both of these forces at bay with anti-inflammatory- and antioxidant-rich foods.

Just as surely as a wide variety of foods can keep inflammation and oxidative stress in check, an even larger group of low-nutrient foods can work to promote these brain-corrosive forces. In a landmark scientific review published in *Obesity Research* in 2009, Australian scientists Garry Egger and John Dixon noted that inflammation-increasing foods "are generally foods or drinks that have been modified, processed or 'value added' in some way, which we have hypothesized are reacted to by the body's immune system as if they were 'foreign invaders.'" For example, diets high in sugar can promote the chronic inflammatory cascade. A can of soda is a prime example of a high-sugar, low-nutrient dietary item; a recent study showed that the level of high-fructose corn syrup found in just a single 8-ounce soda can increase oxidative stress and lower blood antioxidant levels for up to four hours after consumption.

Other components of the typical Western diet, including excess refined carbohydrates, animal fats, and vegetable oils, also run against the health interest of our brain cells. For instance, saturated fats and meat from confined domestic cattle have both been linked to low-grade inflammation in humans. And as important as omega-6 fatty acids are, volumes of international research show that when taken in our current excess, omega-6 oils are well capable of promoting inflammation and oxidative stress. Certainly, the Western diet is attractive to the brain; some scientists, including a group from Scripps Research Institute writing in 2010 in *Nature Neuroscience,* have recently provided evidence that its seductive lure—its sweet, fatty, salty mix—may even be addictive. The toll will be collected in terms of its corrosive force and detrimental influence on nerve cell communication.

## Happy Fats

> Cod-liver oil is valuable because it is a food rather than a
> simple medicament in these cases ... the important place
> the fats hold in the quantitative chemical analysis of the
> human nervous system accounts for their most useful
> dietetic role in melancholic cases.
>
> —*Theodore H. Kellogg, MD, "Dietetics in Mental Diseases," 1887*

Since the early observations of New York psychiatrist Theodore H.
Kellogg, we now have a sophisticated understanding of how different fats affect our nerve cells. The nerve cell coating, scientifically
known as the neuronal membrane, contains a fatty bi-layer that
can become hard and inflexible when it lacks sufficient omega-3
fatty acids. Lack of omega-3 has been associated with changes to
brain physiology and nerve cell structure that are in line with the
changes noted in depression. Excess saturated fats and dietary
cholesterol, combined with our current top-heavy omega-6 intake,
can also disturb the makeup of the lipid bi-layer in the neuronal
membrane. Even miniscule changes to its structure can translate
into compromised signaling between nerve cells. This, depend-
ing on genetic susceptibilities and life stressors, can manifest in
increased risk of depressive symptoms and anxiety.

When omega-3 fatty acids are incorporated into the neuronal membrane, they facilitate optimal signaling both between
and within nerve cells. Omega-3 fatty acids can lower the oxidative stress and inflammation associated with neurological
and psychiatric conditions. In addition, they can promote the
production of the "miracle grow" nerve-supporting BDNF. This
nerve growth factor plays a role in the growth, integrity, and
survival of our nerve cells throughout life. Modern-day fish
oils supplements, and the cod-liver oil advocated by Kellogg,
are rich in omega-3 fatty acids. Recent controlled studies using

fish oil have shown value in some of the most difficult cases of depression—treatment-resistant depression—and also in improving the mental outlook of otherwise healthy adults.

## Dietary Patterns, Depression, and Cognition

In a series of studies that began in the mid-1990s, Dr. Joseph Hibbeln from the U.S. National Institutes of Health observed consistent relationships between higher national fish and seafood consumption and lower relative rates of depression, seasonal affective disorder, bipolar depression, and postpartum depression. Other researchers in the United Kingdom reported that increased annual sugar consumption predicted higher rates of depression. In particular, high levels of soft drink consumption has been linked to depression, psychological distress, and suicidal ideation—after controlling for numerous socioeconomic and lifestyle factors, researchers found that consuming more than half a liter—16 ounces—of soft drinks per day was associated with a 60 percent greater risk of depression.

These early studies opened the door to more detailed investigations into dietary links to depression and cognition. In the years since, a growing number of studies have linked dietary patterns and mood— the results almost exclusively showing that a whole-foods diet closer to nature is protective against depression. Whether the study population involved civil servants from the United Kingdom; healthy women from Baltimore, Maryland; primary care patients from Rochester, Minnesota; pregnant women from Crete, Greece; or randomly chosen adults from Australia's compulsory electoral polls, the results were consistent: intakes of processed meats, fried foods, sugar, refined cereals, and high-fat dairy typically correlated with depression, whereas greater consumption of fish, fruits, vegetables, and whole grains was linked to lower self-reported depressive symptoms. Processed foods and adherence to a Western diet increases the odds of anxiety and depression by about 30 percent, whereas adherence to a high-quality traditional diet decreases the odds by a similar percentage.

In the Baltimore study, women reporting depressive symptoms were 54 percent more likely to be frequent fast-food consumers. In the Rochester Mayo Clinic study, people consuming two to four servings of fruits and vegetables per day were 41 percent less likely to experience frequent mental distress than those consuming one serving or less, and the fruit and vegetable consumption provided better protection against frequent mental distress than did vigorous exercise. When researchers evaluated the dietary patterns of over 500 women during pregnancy, they found that greater adherence to a traditional diet characterized by fish, olive oil, legumes, fruits, vegetables, dairy, and nuts equated to a 50 percent reduction in the risk of postpartum depression (versus those following a Western diet).

Four recent studies from Spain have added value to the mounting evidence, this time using prospective evaluation: taking stock of individual medical history and dietary patterns, and then following those adults for several years. These were not small studies, each one following 10,000 or more young adults for four to six years. The first of the studies showed that adherence to a Mediterranean diet seemed to provide insulation against depression—greater adherence to the diet decreased the risk of clinical depression by 30 percent. Researchers also reported that higher trans-fat intake led to higher odds of depression—a 42 percent increased risk among those with the highest intake of trans-fatty acids. Since trans fats are human-made, synthetic attempts at nutrition, the results fit perfectly with Egger and Dixon's "foreign invader" hypothesis. In another Spanish study involving over 11,000 adults followed for four years, adherence to the Mediterranean diet predicted individual vitality (see the Pursuit of Vitality box below). Most recently, the same group of researchers has reported that after following a group of healthy young adults for six years, results showed that greater adherence to a fast-food diet increased the odds of depression by 36 percent, and the overall intake of commercial baked goods—muffins, donuts, pastries, and so on—was linked to an increased risk of depression.

Similar findings have been noted in the cognitive realm. A number of large population studies in North America and Europe have shown that greater adherence to the Mediterranean diet is associated with protection against cognitive decline in older adults. Researchers in the United Kingdom collected nutritional data provided by mothers and caregivers of 3-year-old children and then followed up with them five and half years later, administering IQ tests to the children, by then aged 8 1/2. Children who had consumed the highest amounts of fatty and sweet processed convenience foods had significantly lower IQ results compared with the children who consumed higher amounts of fish, greens, fruits, vegetables, and grains. Habitual sugar intake and an elevated intake of saturated fats have also been associated with compromised cognitive functioning in healthy adults. Given that low-grade inflammation, even in healthy young adults, is associated with lowered IQ and cognitive abilities, the links between a pro-inflammatory, nature-deficient diet and the loss of cognitive edge should not be surprising.

---

### Dr. Eva's File

Margaret was worried about her son, Jake. At 10 years old, he was having trouble concentrating. He seemed anxious and often depressed. His doctors diagnosed him with ADHD and recommended treating him with medications, but Margaret was concerned about doing so. She came to me asking if there were alternatives. We discussed getting him outdoors—running, exercising, and engaging in creative activities. We also discussed his diet. Jake, like most children his age, preferred junk food. Other than that, being a picky eater, he mostly ate peanut-butter-and-jelly sandwiches, cereal, or pancakes for breakfast, and macaroni and cheese. We then discussed the importance of omega-3 fish oils for brain development and balance, as well as other minerals and vitamins that can be attained from healthy grains, fruits, and vegetables, especially dark leafy greens. Moreover, we talked about the negative effects refined sugar could have on the brain, especially mood and ADHD.

Knowing that it would not be easy, Margaret slowly weaned Jake off processed foods and refined sugars, choosing almond butter over peanut butter and natural sugars like agave syrup. She also attempted to increase his vegetable intake. The improvement in Jake's behavior and mood was remarkable, though there was still room for improvement. And when Jake did eat too much sugar, the difference was definitely noticeable.

> ### Pursuit of Vitality
>
> Although happiness gets lots of attention these days, vitality is an underappreciated asset. Vitality, as defined by psychologists, is emotional strength in the face of internal and external oppositions. It's characterized by living life as an adventure, with excitement and energy, and feeling alive, activated, and enthused. Vitality has been well validated as an excellent marker of both physical and psychological well-being. Roadblocks to vitality include the usual suspects of stress and a sedentary lifestyle. Promoters of vitality include physical fitness, mindful engagement in activities, and connectivity to nature in the physical sense (time spent in nature) and in the nutritional sense (consuming a healthy diet). Adherence to a less-processed diet and/or the consumption of whole foods has been linked to enhanced vitality.

## Bringing Back Nature—Mediterranean or Traditional Diet

Although large population studies provide intriguing information about those who adhere to healthy diets over time, from a scientific perspective we need further details that only so-called intervention studies can provide. Specifically, what happens when we bring individuals back from a processed Western diet and return them to a greater form of nature by switching them to a Mediterranean diet? So far, the answers bode well for mental health and cognition. Switching to the nature-based diet reduces blood markers of inflammation, curbs the spikes of insulin, and pumps up blood levels of antioxidants. Beyond the direct physiological benefits, when otherwise healthy adults adopt a Mediterranean diet, they cut fast-food intake by more than 50 percent.

The brain benefits of a simple short-term switch to a Mediterranean diet were evaluated in a recent study published in a 2011 issue of *Appetite*. Over a 10-day period, a diet higher in fruits, vegetables, fatty fish, low-fat natural dairy, nuts, seeds, and whole-grain cereals (to the exclusion of refined sugar and processed flour, soft drinks, red meats, and prepackaged and processed foods) was shown to improve mental vigor and feelings of alertness and contentment. Compared with the group continuing with the typical Western diet, the nature-diet group showed improvement in some aspects of cognitive functioning as well.

From the name of this diet, you might think that you must dine on Mediterranean food shipped to you at great expense, but this is inaccurate. We prefer calling it a "traditional diet" because the key principles of the Mediterranean diet can largely be replicated with regional fare. Omega-3-rich fish and seafood can be obtained through American and Canadian wild fish, olive trees are now cultivated on this continent, and olive oil is now produced in North America, as are grapes, tomatoes, and whole grains. Locally grown traditional diets, not modified or prepackaged, as close to nature as possible, can return us to a time when we were nutritionally connected to nature.

## Dietary Supplements and the Brain

The shift from whole foods has been accompanied by efforts to reintroduce some elements of nature's nutrients in the form of dietary supplements—over 30,000 types of dietary supplements and counting. Physicians are beginning to embrace some of these dietary supplements, with a recent study showing 72 percent of cardiologists, 66 percent of dermatologists, and 91 percent of orthopedists recommending supplements to their patients. At present, 60 percent of North Americans take some sort of vitamin-based supplement, and about 20 percent consume herb-based products. The emerging research on some of these supplement types—omega-3 fatty acids, various vitamins and minerals, and plant-derived antioxidant/ anti-inflammatory agents in packaged form—is providing encouraging results in the area of mental and cognitive health.

> ### Video Games and Excess Calories
>
> For every hour of daily video game play, a video gamer faces a two-fold increase in the risk of obesity. Beyond simply being a sedentary activity, Canadian researchers have identified an additional video game pathway to obesity. In a study published in 2011 in the *American Journal of Clinical Nutrition*, researchers in Ottawa, Ontario, reported that playing video games for an hour twice per day increases caloric intake. The video gamers consumed 163 extra calories above and beyond any compensation from energy expenditure. The increased food intake occurred regardless of any particular appetite sensations. In separate research published that same year in the *Journal of the American Dietetic Association*, researchers at Dartmouth Medical School found that not only is screen-time snacking frequent but also the top choices are far from broccoli and kale—unhealthy salty and high-sugar choices top the list.

## Supplements and Depression

Controlled studies have shown that the omega-3 fatty acid EPA, or eicosapentaenoic acid, at daily doses between one and two grams, can improve mood in healthy adults, as well as in those suffering from so-called treatment-resistant depression, the most difficult to treat cases. EPA, when added to Prozac, improves outcome by over 30 percent compared with Prozac plus a placebo. Fish oil supplements have also been shown to be helpful for depressive symptoms, learning disorders, and cognition in children. Similar findings have been reported for folic acid and zinc: when these nutrients are added to standard antidepressant medications, the outcome is far better versus the medication plus a placebo. Dozens of studies have shown that low blood levels of zinc, selenium, and B vitamins, particularly folate and B12, are associated with depressive symptoms. Indeed, low blood levels of folate or B12 predict poor outcome in mental health interventions. Patients treated with Prozac who showed low blood folate levels had a 43 percent relapse rate versus a 3 percent relapse in those with the highest blood folate prior to initiating the medication.

Our sun-blocked, nature-deprived indoor lifestyle contributes to lack of vitamin D, a vitamin that influences mood-regulating neurotransmitters. Low levels of vitamin D are associated with risk of major depressive disorder and disturbances to the normal cycles of our body clock. In a double-blind, placebo-controlled study, researchers showed that daily doses of 400 to 800 IU (international units) of vitamin D improved mood during the winter months. Vitamin D significantly influenced aspects of positive affect, including areas involving attention, enthusiasm, motivation, and alertness. Recent controlled studies have shown chromium supplements to be helpful in various aspects of depression, particularly craving for carbohydrates. Lack of magnesium, a mineral we derive from deep green leafy vegetables, has also been linked to depression. When it comes to a simple multivitamin-mineral formula making a difference to mood and cognition in otherwise healthy adults, the research indicates that the very people not taking them, those within the low socioeconomic spectrum, would have the most to gain. And there have also been recent controlled studies suggesting that multivitamin-mineral supplementation can improve fatigue, mood, and cognitive performance in healthy adults enduring high cognitive demands.

## Whole-Food Supplements

In the arena of supplements derived from whole-food sources (i.e., foods or components of foods in powdered form, with water removed), most of the research remains in the experimental stages. Dozens of international studies show that dietary items ranging from apples to turmeric can positively influence behavior in various animal models of chronic stress, depression, and anxiety. There have been human studies showing that cocoa antioxidants, the key components of the cocoa drink consumed by humans for over 3,000 years, can improve memory, reaction time, and other aspects of cognition. Antioxidant components of green tea, another centuries-old beverage linked to protection against depression and cognitive decline, have been shown to improve mood in humans versus placebo capsules. Other small human studies suggest improvement in cognition and mood with antioxidant-rich apple or grape juice. Human studies using actual whole-food supplements are harder to come by, though there has been some research. For example, in a study published in 2004 in the *Canadian Journal of Dietetic Practice and Research*, a blend of 24 plant-derived ingredients, including from green tea, grains, berries, grapes, and sea vegetables, in a product from Genuine Health called greens+ was shown to improve energy and vitality versus placebo in healthy adult women. And recently, melon-derived antioxidants (e.g., in pure calm+ joy, also from Genuine Health) have been shown to improve quality of life, mental outlook, cognitive performance, irritability, and perceptions of stress. The French melons from which the supplement was derived are particularly resilient against spoilage thanks to their high content of the naturally occurring antioxidant superoxide dismutase (SOD). Interestingly, SOD is the very same antioxidant enzyme that works in our defense, and one that is heavily taxed under psychological stress and in mental health disorders. What we are learning from these studies about both individual ingredients and whole-food-derived powdered blends is that nutrition supplementation does matter when it comes to mental health and cognition.

If individual components of a nature-based diet, delivered in supplement form, can provide a mental advantage over placebo, this speaks volumes about what an entire orchestra of whole foods can do for us. At this point we probably don't need any more animal studies showing us that supplemental turmeric can improve depression in animals, that resveratrol from grapes can slow brain aging in mice, or that blueberries can undo cognitive deficits in aged laboratory rats. We have now had over a decade of such reductionist research, and although interesting, the results are often used to infer that there is a single brain food or natural food chemical that can save us from ourselves. The nutritional influences on the brain are extremely complex, and nutrient protectors are emerging as more powerful than the sum of their individual parts. It is becoming clear, as was theorized in the late 1800s, that there is a wide range of brain power foods and that these dietary components work together in orchestral fashion. A transition of research time and resources to clinical intervention studies on whole foods or, at the very least, whole-food supplements, is required. The human studies that do exist clearly tell us that something is wrong with our current dietary patterns.

### Fighting Crime with Food

Peter C. Remondino, vice-president of the California Medical Society, was convinced that crime was influenced, to some degree, by improper diet. Before there were Oprah, Dr. Oz, and over 900 books on amazon.com dedicated to the subject, this American physician wrote extensively on the health properties of the Mediterranean climate and diet. In 1891, a century before it was discovered that supplementing with olive oil may decrease anxiety and promote prosocial behavior, he wrote, "I have no doubt but that if the State would try the experiment . . . the purchase of a few gallons of olive oil would lessen the pressure on Folsom and San Quentin prisons, as well as it would diminish the committals to the Stockton and Napa Asylums."

One hundred years later, Oxford University researchers examined the effects of a daily multivitamin and fish oil combination or two placebos on the behavior of 231 adult offenders. After about four months, there was a 37 percent reduction in serious offenses among the active group (versus a 10 percent reduction in the placebo group). A recent Dutch study involving 221 adult offenders has essentially replicated the findings: a multivitamin and fish oil combination (800 milligrams EPA/DHA) reduced reported offenses by 34 percent among those supplemented, this compared with a 14 percent *increase* in those taking the placebo.

Dr. Joseph Hibbeln of the U.S. National Institutes of Health has reported that nations consuming greater dietary omega-3 fatty acids have lower homicide rates. His follow-up study showed that, in Western nations, homicide rates increased in a linear fashion with mass introductions of linoleic acid. Blood testing has revealed lower levels of omega-3 fatty acids among violent offenders, while in a study of over 3,000 young urban males, low omega-3 intake predicted hostile behavior. Low blood omega-3 levels have also been linked specifically to suicide by violent means.

And then we have sugar. Using data from the 17,000-person British Cohort Study, researchers examined total confectionary intake (i.e., candy) among 10-year-olds. Following up decades later, those children (now 34-year-old adults) who had consumed the highest level of sweets were significantly more likely to have been convicted of a violent offense. The researchers controlled for numerous variables, including family-income level, parenting style, and children's level of education, yet the effect remained.

## Nutri-Ecopsychology

> *Our energy and well-being, physical and mental,*
> *are dependent in the main upon the composition and*
> *quality of the diet. All of it, except fish and other*
> *food taken from the ocean and inland waters, is*
> *derived from the soil, whether in the form of grains,*
> *fruits, or vegetables, or in the form of meat and milk*
> *of animals which, in turn, live upon plant life. Man*
> *must know and respect nature.*
> —National Education Association of the United States, 1951

Ecopsychology is an emerging discipline that views the health of the individual in a context of the health of the planet itself, embracing the notion that the two are inseparable. Nutrition represents a critical component of this field. There are several reasons why ecopsychology might be reframed as nutri-ecopsychology:

- Positive emotions foster environmentally responsible behaviors, and nutritional patterns can influence emotions.
- Nutrition can influence subsequent aspects of ecopsychology even before an individual is born. The foods consumed during pregnancy and lactation can set individual patterns of eating and taste preference, including that geared toward a local traditional diet, for life. In 2010, rather disturbing research showed that the low-grade inflammation produced by the Western diet can have enduring consequences to offspring. Diets high in saturated and trans fats during pregnancy and lactation are associated with subsequent increases in pro-inflammatory chemicals and behavioral changes in infancy and beyond. In other words, we may be giving birth to infants already primed to their own low-grade inflammation, heightened anxiety, and cognitive difficulties. The effects, we are learning, may last through adulthood.
- The direct environmental impact of the Western diet, with all of its processing, sugar additions, heating, and animal-rearing techniques, is like a combine harvester run amok. The Mediterranean diet and local versions of the plant-predominant nature diet have been shown to be far more environmentally friendly. In 2011, the Environmental Working Group made headlines with its Meatless Monday pledge effort—noting that if the U.S. citizenry simply abstained from meat for a single day per week, it would be the environmental equivalent of taking 7.6 million cars off the road.
- Techno-overload, nature withdrawal, and nutrition are not isolated from each other. Spending time in front of the screen has been shown to increase our intake of high-energy, low-nutrient foods and beverages. The ever-present screen is a magnetic lure away from greenspace. Both in the physical and the mindful sense, it takes us away from nature and acts as an obesity provocateur.
- The personal wellness of health-care providers—the individuals who maintain the scaffolding of a healthy person-planet

paradigm—influences their ability to deliver quality care. A 2011 study reports that inadequate workplace nutrition among physicians takes a negative toll on personal wellness *and* professional performance. Clearly, such findings indicate that nutrition is an upstream factor that can facilitate or hinder care of all sorts, including mental health.

---

### Farmed Salmon, Sushi, and the Environment

We have touted the benefits of fish-derived omega-3 fatty acids for brain health, perhaps providing ample justification for a serving of salmon sushi. But a study in the 2009 *Proceedings of the National Academy of Sciences* shows that the farmed-fish industry consumes 88 percent the global fish oil and fish meal produced, and that it takes 11 pounds of wild fish (e.g., anchovies) in feed to yield just 2 pounds of the farmed salmon purchased as sushi. Although farmed salmon has comparable omega-3 levels to wild salmon, it also has much higher levels of omega-6, the fat we are overconsuming. This is an important point in nutri-ecopsychology—lowering the overall dietary omega-6 intake to resemble intake in the early 20th century helps to cause a relative increase in omega-3 levels without putting pressure on global fish stocks. Moreover, there are ongoing concerns with the environmental toxins PCBs in farmed fish. Canadian and Alaskan canned wild salmon may be a better option, as long as it remains sustainable.

Visit www.seachoice.org for more information.

---

## The High Cost of the Western Diet

If viewed strictly from an economic price point, the Western diet is cheap. An individual can purchase 1,500 calories for around $5 at fast-food and convenience stores. Viewed only as a source of caloric energy, the cost of potato chips is 80 percent less than a raw carrot. North Americans, especially those in low socioeconomic brackets who cannot afford the "insurance policy" of dietary supplements, are encouraged to eat healthier fare, yet they are expected to pay more to do so. Chronic illness, mental health in particular, can drain financial and physical energy resources, making convenient and inexpensive calories look even more attractive and creating something of a vicious cycle.

Economics aside, we are paying an untold environmental price in our system of confining animals and attempting to grow them rapidly with foods foreign to their natural diets, while at the same time strip-mining nutrients off food and then adding some of them back in as we try to dress up overly processed food for consumers. Candy-like cereals provide a prime example of a highly processed food made to look attractive by the addition of what amounts to a multivitamin.

Numerous media articles on the popularity and increase in consumption may inadvertently give rise to the perception that organic foods are now taking over North American shelves. But this is far from reality. Although organic foods have grown in popularity, particularly among the affluent, 96 percent of retail food sales are of nonorganic foods. Before we can even imagine organic foods going mainstream, at least in a legitimate sense, the price disparity needs to be fixed. The high price of organic food currently acts as a deterrent. We also need to mend the disconnect between people and the agribusinesses that serve up food. Big food is a sort of Wizard of Oz behind the curtain, happy to keep the status quo and serve up the Western diet, with all of its environmental consequences, to an unknowing public. Despite a sprinkling of exposé documentaries such as *We Feed the World* and *Food, Inc.,* research shows that the public does not know, or doesn't want to know, what goes on behind that curtain.

## Eating Right for Your Brain—and the Planet

Although the situation may seem bleak, a sense of optimism should prevail. The solutions to these problems are complex, yet connectivity to nature and a greater connection to the naturalness of dietary items, foods in their whole-food form, appear to short-circuit the lure of convenience. Optimistically, for over 50 percent of U.S. food shoppers, convenience might be trumped by considerations such as taste, freshness, health aspects, food safety, and the organic nature of food. In addition, a 2011 report by McGill University researchers in *Appetite* indicates that the craving for highly palatable, nature-deprived foods can be cut off by visualizing nature scenes or being in nature. Taking a nature break from the screen, perhaps even a few mindful minutes gazing through a window at nature or interacting with an animal, might help break the cycle of craving.

Farmers' markets and community- and school-based gardens are gaining momentum, helping to put a dent in the broad divides between people, agriculture, and food. Across hundreds of North American university campuses, sustainable food projects are influencing young minds. As Dr. Peggy Barlett, an anthropologist at Emory University in Atlanta, GA, contends, these efforts are incubators for broad change. Sustainable catering, consisting of foods close to nature, seasonal and local where possible, is a practice gaining a strong foothold. Corporations are starting to wise up to the fact that a cart full of glazed donuts wheeled into the mid-morning meeting room is not compatible with so-called green and sustainable agendas for which they claim to stand.

Even more encouragement comes from the first (in 2010) of what will be an ongoing international Healthy Agriculture, Healthy Nutrition, Healthy People conference. The conference garnered international attention thanks to its high-profile scientific collaboration and representation from numerous nations, and its mission dedicated to the notion that ecology, psychology, nutrition, food supply, and urban planning are intertwined as parts of the whole. As the organizing committee stated, "In promoting healthy agriculture, healthy nutrition, healthy people, we are in fact promoting a single integrated model...not three independent concepts or goals, but rather integral parts of the whole that support and sustain a healthy society and environment."

Positive steps are being made in dismantling the relationships between governments, professional dietetic groups, and the companies that otherwise influence each other in pushing the environmental toxin known as the Western diet. Potential conflicts of interest among these groups abound, and rational food scientists are finding them increasingly intolerable. Concerned members within the American Dietetic Association have formed their own Hunger and Environmental Nutrition Practice Group, distancing themselves from big food. A push-back is occurring, one that in many ways resembles the very early days of the tobacco resistance. Just a few decades ago, when half of North American adults smoked, it might have seemed like an impossible public health task to cut smoking rates. Although smoking rates remain too high, they are 50 percent lower than they once were, underscoring the notion that change is possible in a relatively short period. When people become personally involved in the development and production of even a few homegrown items, they begin to have an appreciation of the concept of naturalness and will be more likely to query the operations behind the agribusiness curtain. There is a small opening in that curtain right now, and a growing segment of the food-consuming audience is beginning to see that there is no wizard; rather, there are smoke and mirrors, actors, and people pulling strings and swinging spotlights, together running the show known as the Western diet. While the show goes on, people and planet are both enduring a low-grade inflammation. Nutrition represents a pivot between ecology and psychology, a potential safe passage out or one that can take us toward a more dangerous backdraft. Encouraging a more mindful understanding of how dietary choices impact ecology and psychology, fostered through contact with and concern for nature, can help douse these flames of inflammation that are making us and our planet unwell.

# 9
CHAPTER

# *Vis Medicatrix Naturae:* The Healing Power of Nature and Ecotherapy

*What then do I mean tonight by the healing power of nature? I mean to refer to the way in which Nature ministers to our minds, all more or less diseased by the rush and racket of civilization, and helps to steady and enrich our lives. My first point is that there are deeply-rooted, old established, far-reaching relations between Man and Nature which we cannot ignore without loss . . . there would be less "psychopathology of everyday life" if we kept up our acquaintance . . . we have put ourselves beyond a very potent vis medicatrix if we cease to be able to wonder at the grandeur of the star-strewn sky, the mystery of the mountains, the sea eternally new, the way of the eagle in the air, the meanest flower that blows, the look in a dog's eye.*

—Professor J. Arthur Thomson, "Vis Medicatrix Naturae," keynote address at the annual meeting of the British Medical Association, 1914

Observations and discussions of the healing power of nature, in Latin *vis medicatrix naturae,* can be traced back to Hippocrates and his position that "nature is the physician of diseases." There are countless interpretations of the meaning of *vis medicatrix naturae,* and the debates are clouded by the complex definitions of the word "nature" itself. Although many concede that *vis medicatrix naturae* can be amplified by external factors, it has typically been defined as an internal healing response written into our DNA. Consider, for example, the way in which a cut on the skin repairs itself. We favor the alternate and more literal interpretation of Professor J. Arthur Thomson: the healing power of nature is associated with mindful immersion in and contact with the natural portions of our external world. In our text we also define nature as the nonbuilt, nonsynthetic environment, with its sights, sounds, aromas, plants, animals, and unseen medicinal agents. And if, as Hippocrates supposed, nature is indeed the physician of disease, we must be concerned when that physician becomes unwell and suffers burnout, as many health-care providers and caregivers do. The record shows that our planet physician, the natural world, is becoming unwell: it is showing the signs of burnout.

Ecopsychiatry and ecopsychology are shedding light on the mental connection to environmental collapse in this situation and providing solutions. Collectively, the mental-health-care researchers and clinicians within these professions recognize that the health of humans and the planet are entirely interdependent. Physicians and allied health-care professionals of all types are beginning to embrace ecotherapy, an umbrella term for the practical application of a bimodal approach to brain health. On the one side of the ecotherapy coin is mindful nature interaction; on the other side is a commitment to nature through environmental awareness and understanding.

Ecotherapy requires mindfulness, not simply a contrived get-back-to-nature effort without conscious thought. Although contact with nature may have antidepressant and antianxiety effects akin to some psychotropic medications, it's essential to recognize that nature cannot be abused or taken for granted, and that humans can benefit from it only so long as they truly care for it. Environmental awareness in the ecotherapeutic sense goes beyond recycling cans and carrying an eco–tote bag. Although they are important contributions, a much greater depth is required if *vis medicatrix naturae* is to continue. The ecotherapeutic system is not a matter of taking a few pictures of the Rocky Mountains with a bamboo wood–encased "green" smartphone and then motoring on to Vegas. As environmental studies expert Dr. Robert Michael Pyle states, "If people feel that they are discharging their responsibility as conservationists by sleeping twice on their sheets in a premium hotel, the overall effect could be counterproductive."

Being in and around nature can have a medicinal effect, yet we can elevate the benefits through a conscious interaction with the natural world. The good news is that truly getting in contact with nature—powering down the gadgets and becoming mindfully engaged and emotionally rejuvenated in nature's presence—cultivates a greater depth of environmental concern. Ecotherapeutic prescriptions, such as a prescription for green exercise, will feed forward the concern for greenspace and the overall health of the environment in a mutually beneficial continuous loop.

As we also discuss below, the skills of a good clinician can be amplified by the direct environmental influence of *vis medicatrix naturae* in outdoor settings. It is now becoming clear that greenspace may be the ideal setting for enhancing therapeutic outcomes when the mental-health-care provider conducts sessions within natural settings. Finally, here in our concluding chapter we come full circle on the technology discussions of Chapter 1, wading into the murky waters of virtual nature, the structural premise being that microchip-delivered nature, plastic trees, and more screens are an eco-solution to our nature deprivation.

## Ecopsychology in North America—What Took So Long?

Reaching into the archives of North American medical history, we found numerous quotes from distinguished physicians and scientists that might be interpreted as an enduring and widespread recognition that nature contact has medicinal properties. They might also be interpreted as widespread acceptance of the notion that the turn from nature—indeed, the destruction of nature and introduction of the synthetic—was not without mental health consequence.

In 1875, physician Franklin B. Hough addressed the American Public Health Association, stating that both the preservation of primeval forests and the cultivation of new forest growth was in the best interest of public health because of "the cheerful and tranquilizing influence which they exert upon the mind, more especially when worn down by mental labor, or convalescent from sickness." Thomson, in his 1914 "Vis Medicatrix Naturae" address, stated that "in a period of evolution which has been mainly urban, we miss our contact with nature—most of all, perhaps, in youth, for it remains true of the child who goes forth every day, that what he sees becomes part of him for a day or for a year, or for stretching cycles of years." One year later, New York psychiatrist Albert W. Ferris addressed the annual meeting of the American Medico-Psychological Association, maintaining that the state should continue to be diligent in its conservation of the Saratoga Springs area: "Sylvan streams, banks of ferns, limpid pools, sandy stretches, shady dells and sunny nooks combine to provide variety and interest, and to lead the often irritable or unhappy patient out of his mood into one of placidity and content, and into an enjoyment of existence."

Dr. Lester K. Ade, superintendent of Pennsylvania public schools, was concerned with the dual problem of suboptimal doses of nature for children and the issues of environmental destruction. In 1937 he wrote, "Many of the natural facilities for using leisure time such as forests, rivers and fields have suffered somewhat from destruction, pollution and congestion, as a result of modern developments in industry . . . the stress of modern life has driven our youth and adults to create artificial amusements. The almost universal recourse to these artificial forms of amusement is a result of two principal circumstances; first, the inaccessibility of natural leisure activities, and second, the promise of profit for those who provide the commercial forms of entertainment."

Interrelated matters of conservation, technology, canned forms of amusement, dwindling contact with nature, a frightening future of nature deprivation among our youth, and the overall mental health implications—all of it was being discussed by doctors, educators, and scientists for the better part of a century. However, without scientific credibility, they remained discussions only, and as psychiatry and psychology galvanized into legitimate scientific professions, the notion of *vis medicatrix naturae,* at least in its natural, green context, was quickly disappearing in the rearview mirror. For professions seeking scientific credibility, such soft notions would be best swept into the dustbin of history. One of the founding fathers of North American psychology, Columbia University professor Edward Thorndike, had no time for any talk or teaching of emotional connections to the nonhuman inhabitants of the natural world, referring to the love of plants as "unreasonable and mischievous idolatry" and stating firmly that animals are "utterly unaffected by the feelings we may have toward them." He scorned physicians who identified themselves as naturalists in their writings, stating that they psychologize "about animals as a lover might psychologize about his beloved." Thorndike, who would influence generations of psychologists, stated, "The boy who collects moths, who steals birds' eggs, who pokes the unlucky crab over onto its back and in fascination watches his uncomfortable efforts to right himself, who takes his toy animals apart to put them together again, is nearer the scientific pathway than the noble product of sentimental nature-study who loves the worms and cares for the dear plants."

With very few exceptions, following Thorndike's assertions, there would be decades of silence related to the importance of our emotional connection to plants and animals in the context of positive mental health and to the idea that animals and plants are utterly affected by the feelings we have toward them. Our feelings toward them determine their very fate, which, in turn, influences ours. It would take psychologists and psychiatrists decades before they would begin to galvanize into action with the realization that nature has a medicinal influence and that in the girl or boy who righted Thorndike's overturned crab, showing empathy toward its struggle, there might be a pathway toward scientific salvation of the planet. Of the few prominent psychiatrists who did speak up, J. Berkeley Gordon and Karl Menninger in the United States and William C. Gibson in Canada were among the most notable. Their comments are noteworthy because they were bold enough to make them at a time when pharmaceutical companies were becoming the guiding lights of psychiatry. Green talk was considered unscientific and far from the forefront of discussions within psychiatric and psychological organizations

In his 1952 piece entitled *The Psychiatric Values of Wilderness,* Gordon captured the very essence of the two-way street of ecotherapy— a cost-effective means of nature immersion as preventive medicine for mental health, with an appreciation of the vulnerability of nature itself: "It is a lot pleasanter, and a lot cheaper, to prevent these [mental health] ailments and even cure them in their early stages by getting back at regular intervals to the peace and quiet of the tall trees, the lakes and rivers, the mountains of our wilderness areas, rather than wait until a real mental illness develops . . . We have been short-sighted and wasteful because our natural resources seemed inexhaustible. But they are not!"

Menninger wrote extensively on the subject of environmental influences on mental health, and in 1959 his work was submitted to the U.S. Congress debating the planned National Wilderness Act. He wrote, "Another psychological need is for the maintenance of contact with nonhuman nature. The simplest way, perhaps, is through pets . . . add the somewhat artificial but pleasant provisions in an accessible and properly maintained park—trees, flowers, shrubs, lawns, lakes, and streams. In my opinion, we must add to this a proximity to larger non-urban areas of farm or wilderness or near-wilderness as essential to the mental health of both child and adult." Discussing the lack of planning and its effects on people, he stated, "Part of this failure is a lack of vision on the part of their predecessors. They didn't see that we would need ten times as many national parks as we have. They waited until now to establish wilderness areas . . . they failed to give us one tenth the area of city parks that we need. They forgot that privacy was just as important as social contact for each individual."

In 1965, University of British Columbia psychiatrist and professor of neurological sciences William C. Gibson presented a lecture entitled "Wilderness—a Psychiatric Necessity," in which he underscored the need for conservation of wilderness and cultivation of parks: "There is no doubt in my mind, as a psychiatrist, about these positive medical values. The parks of London were once called 'the lungs of the people.' Today, we should be shouting from the rooftops that the parklands of America are the greatest mental health guardians we have."

Finally, in the early 1970s, a small group of psychologists and psychiatrists began to kindle the modern ecopsychiatry and ecopsychology movements. The first ecopsychiatry workshop was held at the American Psychiatric Association's 1974 annual meeting. Attendance was encouraged under the following event description, "Population growth, pollution, and the experience of inadequate environmental resources affect quality of life, mental health, and the nature of human interactions. The body of knowledge of psychiatric disturbances caused by human interference with planetary housekeeping— ecology—will be discussed as well as ecopsychiatric methodology in tracing the etiology of psychopathology to environmental factors."

Psychiatric disturbances caused by humans interfering with planetary housekeeping? At last we were getting somewhere! New Jersey psychiatrist Dr. Aristide H. Esser, the organizer of this and other ecopsychiatry symposiums that would follow at the World Mental Health Congress meetings, defined the work: "The ecopsychiatrist attends to the psychiatric symptomatology caused by derailments in the man-environment relations. In this endeavor he must use multidisciplinary insights necessary for the reordering of the mind and the ordering of the environment."

Around the same time, European psychologists coined the term "ecopsychology" and described their own focus on the interactions between human mental health, contemporary ecological problems, and the budding efforts toward conservation. In addition, decades before the Internet and smartphones, German ecopsychologists Lenelis Kruse and Carl Graumann predicted that "the near omnipresence of computers and the invasion by new and more media" would create fertile ground for informational overload and a magnetic lure to sources of screen-based entertainment. These European ecopsychologists were ahead of the curve. The entire package of technological overload and environmental pressures, they felt, would have tremendous relevance to personal mental health and psychology as a profession. They were right, and as they introduced the ecopsychology concept to North American psychologists in the 1980s, it provided much-needed sparks to the kindling of professional interest. Slowly and surely, writings and conferences on ecopsychology and ecotherapy expanded. Still, the concept was far from an overnight sensation, and it wouldn't be until 2009 that the first peer-reviewed journal *Ecopsychology* would make its debut. It has often been said within the scientific community that, within the sciences, in the absence of an institutionalized journal, the discipline doesn't exist.

So, here we are, at the infancy of a movement, a still-fledgling operation that should have had massive, across-the-board professional support decades ago. Mental-health-care providers are not solely in the business of addressing existing psychopathology; they are much more broadly the professional guides to positive mental health and the gatekeepers of preventive medicine. The teachings of psychiatry and psychology are powerful additions to public and planetary health; they matter to all of us. Indirectly, they have tremendous influence on the day-to-day practice and lifestyle advice provided by other frontline health defenders, family doctors in particular. The low-grade inflammation of a disturbed natural environment is presenting itself as a low-grade inflammation in humans—it is becoming more broadly accepted that the high rates of obesity, stress, and mental health disorders are being experienced by the canaries in the postindustrial environmental coalmine. Australian preventive medicine expert Garry Egger has stated that we have spent our time and resources on noble efforts to resuscitate the canary, while paying no mind to cleaning out the mine shaft.

The burning question is, what took us so long? The quotations we provide above illustrate that the advocates, those with an early recognition of the interrelatedness of environmental stewardship and mental health, were vocal, yet somehow stifled. A few suspects for the squandered time could be rounded up: political and financial motives, overconfidence in technology, reductionist scientific approaches, pharmaceutical fondness, the view that science and empathy are distinct, and profit-driven commercial interests that guide our information overload and the perceived notion that in omnipresent screens and synthetic means of entertainment lies the key to happiness. These same forces are still at play, arguably stronger than ever. Recent advancements in the field of ecopsychology are encouraging, but it would be naive to think that everything has been sorted and that there is no risk of regression to a place of professional and personal complacency. We are presuming that psychiatrists spend time engaging in talk therapy with patients, yet the research shows a massive decline in such therapy in the last decade. Moreover, the recent interest in ecopsychology may unwittingly give the impression that an army of consumer psychologists—the folks who teach corporations how to get you to consume nature-deprived food, chemical-laden goods, and dumpsters full of other stuff you probably don't need—have indeed closed up shop.

---

### Using Nature as a Retail Venus Flytrap

Just as surely as there are now concerned psychologists and behavioral scientists working to conserve nature and enhance the human-planet health paradigm, there are some who see a different sort of opportunity in the way the brain is influenced by nature. Psychologists are often paid handsome sums to align marketing strategists with the goal of maximizing consumption. Retail settings are inherently depressing: large studies comparing rates of depression and land use have indicated that beyond the built environment per se, the percentage of retail availability increases the odds of depression. Parking lots in a neighborhood are a surrogate marker of retail land use, and an increase of them is associated with social isolation. On the upside, the presence of greenery mitigates the negative relationship between retail land use and depression.

Superficially, it makes sense to dress up retail settings with greenery. Marketing experts are uncomfortable with the prospect of losing retail sales if consumers are not in the right mood, and for years they have tried countless environmental tricks to increase mood-related consumption—lighting, aromas, music, colors, and so on.

In 2007, Dr. Renate Buber of the Vienna University of Economics and Business Administration discovered what might be a dark side to so-called evolutionary store design, which is retail design that introduces natural elements—water, plants, animals. Surely, this would be a good thing. What happens, though, when that evolutionary store design is adjacent to a fast-food outlet? Buber and colleagues measured consumer patterns in a mall for 56 days, manipulating the evolutionary variable via the presence of water, plants, and artificial animals (versus the control of wooden pillars). The nature elements did everything a marketer would want them to do: they slowed down the pace of the shoppers, made them stay longer in that particular area, and most importantly, significantly increased sales at the fast-food outlet. Studies are underway to evaluate the effect of virtual plants and water as a way to promote further consumption. In the meantime, consumers should be cognizant of what might sit behind, or adjacent to, these manufactured vistas.

## The Doctor Is In—a New Psychotherapy Office

Ecopsychology's message of humanity's interconnectedness with nature has led some mental health providers not only to prescribe nature therapy but also to take their own practice into the great outdoors. This may include a garden setting outside the therapist's office, though increasingly it involves meeting at designated parks, arboretums, botanic gardens, or urban greenspace. The benefits of wilderness and other natural settings have been described as helpful in group psychotherapy since the 1950s—these were often incorporated into the camp therapy—and the approach is now being used for individual counseling.

In a study published in *Psychiatry Investigation* in 2009, researchers reported on the one-month treatment of 63 patients with moderate to severe depression. Patients had been assigned to once-weekly cognitive-behavioral therapy in either a hospital setting or a forest setting (an arboretum), and a third control group was treated using standard outpatient care in the community. The overall depressive symptoms were reduced most significantly in the forest group, and the odds of complete remission were relatively high—20 to 30 percent higher than that typically observed from medication alone. Moreover, the individuals whose therapy was conducted in a forest setting had more pronounced reductions in physiological markers of stress, including lower levels of the stress hormone cortisol and improvements in heart rate variability, a marker of dominance of the "rest and digest" (parasympathetic) branch of the nervous system. The researchers concluded that the psychotherapy settings are not merely places; they can become part of the therapy itself. The results lend credence to *vis medicatrix naturae* and support the claims of ecotherapists already conducting psychotherapy in natural settings.

Weather permitting, counseling sessions in natural environments offer additional benefits beyond the mood-regulating and cognitive-enhancing effects of greenspace. Reducing stress enhances cognitive function, and the direct ability of natural settings to lessen attentional fatigue amplifies what a skilled therapist has to offer. Patients may also benefit from physical activity, say, if the session allows for walking. The natural setting may allow for expanded opportunities for practical mindfulness, meditation, and other mind-body techniques before, during, or after the counseling session. On top of this, some individuals appreciate that they do not have to walk into a building with pronounced signage confirming that they are indeed seeing a mental-health-care provider. Counseling in greenspace, taking on the appearance of walking and talking with a friend, is not a panacea that will undo the stigma that acts as a primary barrier to accessing mental health care. However, given the staggeringly low levels of mental-health-care use among those in need, if even a small degree of comfort is provided by having some of the sessions out-of-office, a meaningful difference might be made.

## Vitamin G Prescriptions—Forest, not Pharmacy

For the last 40 years, nutrition dictionaries have formally listed vitamin G as an obsolete name for riboflavin, or vitamin B2. However, in 2006, Dutch health scientist Dr. Peter P. Groenewegen and colleagues reinvented "vitamin G" as a now widely used reference to the medicinal influence of greenspace. Primary care doctors, psychiatrists, and other mental health providers are now beginning to write formal prescriptions for vitamin G, with specified amounts of exercise and/or time spent in urban greenspace, gardens, arboretums, and forests. Research shows that stressed adults may actually need that vitamin G prescription in hand: those under stress have the most to gain from vitamin G; however, they are the least likely to make their way to the greenspace dispensary unless they have guidance.

The savviest prescribers are providing specific prescriptions: walking, hiking, gardening, and opportunities for solitude and contemplation in green locations. Vitamin G prescriptions are usually served up with instructions on mindfulness, underscoring that the benefits of time spent in nature are amplified if the individual is *there* in the true sense of the word: strolling through a park while engaged with a smartphone screen may cause a vitamin G deficiency.

## Plastic Trees and Plasma Screens—Providing Communion with Nature?

In the 1970s, it was suggested that plastic trees might be an economical trade-off as a means of conserving nature. Although plastic trees couldn't proactively clean the air, they might make people feel content, acting as a sort of societal pacifier that would, in turn, take financial pressure off the need to maintain areas of actual nature. In 1973, American urban planner Martin H. Krieger claimed in the prestigious journal *Science* that technology could easily be applied to the manufacture of artificial wilderness areas, noting that "much more can be done with plastic trees and the like to give most people the feeling that they are experiencing nature." The plastics industry was certainly in a position to oblige, tickled with the imagery of plastic bamboo gardens and giant PVC sequoias in all downtown metro areas. After all, this was an influential urban planner talking, and not merely about dressing up store windows; this was plastic on a grand scale. Ecologists, predictably, were having none of it—in particular Dr. Hugh H. Iltis, who responded that there should be widespread reading of Krieger's article, if only so that people can "catch a glimpse of the nightmare future that technology is preparing for man and nature . . . What if, long after all of nature has finally been ground up in the garbage disposal of the technologic sink, it becomes clear that there are indispensable genetic needs for many of these components of nature?"

The strong rebukes by naturalists and ecology scientists have done nothing to stop the fascination with plastic cases and silicon chips as a means of keeping us content, wrapped up in the feel-good packaging of environmental conservation. The logic of keeping people away from actual nature by giving them plastic and virtual nature as a way to protect the environment is fantasy in itself. The fallacy of the plastic argument is exposed by the numerous research studies showing that lifetime contact with actual nature is the greatest stimulator of pro-environmental behaviors and concerns for nature welfare. The same is true of the rejoicing in the fact that annual visits to national and state parks are down, another fallacious conclusion that fewer people in such places contributes broadly to nature conservation. How absurd! A true cause for celebration would be news reports of more people entering national parks, or even better, local urban forests and greenspace, with the right amount of, as Aldo Leopold called it, "perception"—his term for mindfulness. As he said, "The outstanding characteristic of perception is that it entails no consumption and no dilution of any resource. The swoop of the hawk, for example, is perceived by one as the drama of evolution . . . to promote perception is the only truly creative part of recreational engineering."

Obviously, we don't need more people traveling great distances, only to chew up the terrain, and we certainly don't need noisy tourists raising the stress hormone levels of animals when they fly by on an overhead mission to get a trophy photograph. However, we do need more people making mindful contact with nature. Some of the greatest maneuvers in North American nature conservation have been accomplished by people who were inspired to act after personal experiences in local and national natural areas. If the national parks experienced a massive uptick in visits, as occurred in the 1950s, the onus would be on us to manage that properly, to inspire and educate, and to do whatever we could to nurture meaningful connectivity to nature within those visits. Of critical importance is that the visits be used as a springboard to the mindful awareness of the importance of local greenspace treasures. It can be done: we are well capable of establishing and supporting a proper balance in local and national nature contact and conservation. The answer is not to discourage nature contact by posting a societal Keep Off the Grass! sign. Nor do the solutions reside in better use of screensavers or more picnics under a collection of mobile phone towers dressed up as pine trees. As Dr. Robert Michael Pyle says, "What is the extinction of a condor or an albatross to a child who has never known a wren? Shallow contact with nature leads to shallow solutions for conservation." A century and a half earlier, in 1848, Henry David Thoreau said it a different way: "Talk of mysteries! Think of our life in nature—daily to be shown matter, to come in contact with it—rocks, trees, wind on our cheeks! the solid earth! the actual world! the common sense! Contact! Contact!"

Since children spend lots of time on the Internet, and nearly 100 percent of North American schools use the Internet in education, it might be easy to presume that the physical nature withdrawal could be compensated for by using this access to increase awareness of conservation and biodiversity issues. So far that hasn't worked out too well. When querying children about conservation knowledge and animal protection, researchers have found that Google media content is shaping these children's brains with a bias toward the exotic animals (the giant panda, for instance) and away from the more important aspects of local biodiversity. Lost is the knowledge and willingness to protect a broad variety of species that exist right in their backyards and gardens, the species that children should be making contact with. This is troubling, since individuals have far more influence over local biodiversity than they do over an exotic animal several continents away. School administrators cannot sit back and let the Internet dictate such critical aspects of environmental education. As the researchers of the study published in 2011 in *PLoS ONE* conclude, "Our study simply adds another call to push the children outside and away from the screens." A study evaluating the effects of virtual nature on attitudes toward preservation of natural areas indicates that the highly selective presentation of nature scenes by the commercial media and simulated nature experiences involving scenes highly rated for beauty (i.e., picturesque equivalents of the exotic giant panda) cause a decline in support for the acquisition and preservation of local natural areas. But virtual reality is not reality; indeed, it has been more aptly described as hyperreality—and therein may lie the problem. Its brilliance, glamour, and beauty are maximized, so only the giant panda and Lake Louise make the cut, while everything else fades in comparison. Local doesn't just take a backseat—it gets kicked out of the car.

Our issue is not with the efficacy of virtual nature in mental health but, rather, with the unintended consequences—and there are always unintended consequences with technology. Much like with plastic trees, it becomes difficult to dismiss the direct environmental fallout from using screen-based gadgets as a nature surrogate; gadgets are, after all, energy consumers and they include precious parts that require mining. Consider that smartphones consume three and a half times more energy than standard phones. The individual contribution of mobile phones may not seem like much—the equivalent of driving a vehicle just a few extra hours per year—until you consider that there are 5 billion in use. The overall information/communications technology footprint is, incredibly, on par with global air travel. It has been estimated that, unless things change, we will have to build 200 additional nuclear power plants in the next 15 to 20 years just to accommodate the energy-consumption needs of our gadgets alone.

We have no doubt that simulated nature can have medicinal effects, and while these may not be as strong as nature in its complete form, the scientific evidence supporting isolated elements of nature does exist. Without question, some of the research we discussed in the earlier chapters involved stress reduction and cognitive enhancement upon viewing photographic and video-based scenes of natural environments. We acknowledge that natural light boxes, dawn stimulators, acoustic gadgets with the sounds of crickets and birds, negative ion generators, and aromatherapy devices are just some of the examples of manufactured nature with medicinal potential. Indeed, sitting in a virtual forest has been shown to reduce stress, although in head-to-head duals, actual nature experience appears to have the edge on mental energy, vitality, and restoration. Actual nature enhances a positive mood state, leads to greater reflection, and improves our ability to work through life problems more effectively than does virtual nature.

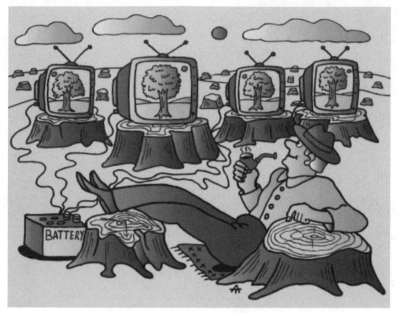

In a study published in 2008 in the *Journal of Environmental Psychology*, 90 young adults were split into three groups and asked to complete a series of complex and stressful cognitive tasks for 30 minutes. There was one significant environmental variable that was changed among the groups: a window view to a nature scene; the same window view to a nature scene except it was presented on a wall-mounted, high-definition, flat-screen plasma TV of similar size to the window; or a blank wall. Lighting level was kept constant for each group. The groups each had a five-minute waiting period before and after the cognitive tasks, during which the participants could freely gaze. The actual window view held the participants' attention longer than did the same view depicted on a plasma screen, and physiological markers of stress showed the greatest recovery in the group that viewed the actual nature scene outside the window versus either the plasma TV set or the blank wall. The plasma TV was better than a blank wall, but not as good as a view of nature impeded by only a thin pane of glass.

Environmental issues aside, the technological co-opting of nature may be establishing an adaptation in us, particularly in our youth, that is not altogether healthy. As younger generations grow up on plastic and plasma nature, they can become oblivious to what once was, and the fallout from *not* having what once was in nature can influence countless outcomes, from conservation to stress reduction. Moreover, if individual aspects of manufactured nature—photographic images, negative ions generated from a machine, or aromatherapy administered via a steamer—can have such medicinal effects when alone, what might be the effects of losing very broad aspects of nature as it was once known generations ago? In truth, younger generations set a new baseline norm for the environment, and lack of a comparative baseline from the experience of "what once was" sets the stage for, as University of Washington technology–nature–human interaction expert Dr. Peter H. Kahn calls it, "environmental generational amnesia." Virtual nature ultimately "grows" to become normal. It can indeed help us to some degree, and combined with a lack of appreciation of what once was, it masks the severity of environmental problems. If we are going to start taking virtual nature to the places that technology can surely take it, we must consider the massive consequences. Kahn and his colleagues said it best: "For example, if you try to explain to a person what we, as humans, are missing in terms of the fullness of the human relation with nature, a well-meaning person can look at you blankly and respond, 'but I don't think we're missing anything.' It is hard enough to address environmental problems, such as global climate change when people are aware of them; it becomes all the harder when they are not."

Well-intentioned scientists, with assistance from military and space programs, are hard at work developing state-of-the-art virtual nature experiences. Undoubtedly, they will succeed in their efforts at replicating, as closely as possible, every dynamic aspect of nature—sounds, scents, weather, clouds, and much more. Even as they work exhaustively on virtual nature technology, other scientists are, refreshingly, fully aware of the dilemma this might present. On the one hand, it would be ideal for the elderly, the hospitalized, the traumatized, the isolated (e.g., in space, at sea, or in the Arctic), and other selective uses. On the other hand, it might make people less conscious of environmental issues and lead to less time outdoors and a diminished connectivity to nature. We would suggest that, as the research stands, the broad use of extreme virtual nature devices—hyperreality—has the potential to cause broad societal and planetary harm in the form of unintended consequences.

---

### Biodiversity for Brain Health

A century ago, New York psychiatrist Albert W. Ferris held that the mentally therapeutic influence of nature was in its variety. Writing in 1916 in the journal *Modern Hospital,* he stated that people are often affected by environmental details that are out of conscious awareness. In discussing hospital and sanatorium greenspace, he urged landscape gardeners to include variety in planting, maintain preservation of wild features already present (rock outcroppings and vines), and avoid what he called the "deformity of uniformity." Recently at the University of Sheffield, Professor Richard A. Fuller and colleagues found that the mental health benefits of 15 urban greenspace settings were positively associated with a greater richness of plant and bird species. Biodiversity was a variable in the ability of natural settings to influence mental well-being.

Researchers at Charles Sturt University in Albury, Australia, have extended these results, reporting in 2011 that even after controlling a range of variables, well-being within urban neighborhoods was associated with species variety, abundance of local birds, and totality of vegetation cover. Of course, more research is needed before we can conclude that deficiencies in biodiversity *cause* direct changes to mental outlook. However, it does lend support to the theory of an innate connection to nature and helps to guide priorities in conservation. The findings indicate that we need to consider the conservation of plant and animal life

---

> within urban and suburban settings on an equal plane with that
> of our national parks and wilderness areas. Giant sequoias and
> giant pandas get well-deserved attention, yet local shrubs and
> birds, even insects, are no less important to the health of humans
> and the planet.

## The Leisure Problem and Nature Identity

When mental health experts are queried on ways in which to reduce stress, many offer solutions related to use of leisure time—exercise being the prime example. In many ways, our spare time is either for or against us when it comes to health. What we do with our time out of work, academic, and family obligations is vital, and the American Psychiatric Association recognized this when it convened its Committee on Leisure Time and Its Uses in the 1960s. The chair of that committee, Dr. Alexander Reid Martin, concluded that mental-health-care providers would increasingly turn their attention to a population that was leisure stricken—the population needed serious guidance in the proper use of leisure time. Leisure was defined as a state of mind, one with the capacity for play, wondering, marveling, attending, reflecting, meditating, looking, listening, and relaxing of the whole person. He was describing mindfulness. Leisure was everything that idle time wasn't; leisure should be as restorative as sleep. Martin suggested that people were actually working to escape confrontation with leisure in the mindful sense. There might be some physical health benefits; however, they were considered only mechanical acts unless they were conducted in the proper state of mind. Long before screens would fully extend their powerful reach, Martin was worried about squandered leisure time and did not see a bright future for those people who remained unfit for leisure, surmising that they would "exist as sterile robots, alienated from life and from themselves, living vicariously and so deadened that they compulsively seek overstimulation from the extreme, the lurid, the bizarre, and the macabre."

Given the popularity of violent video games as a leisure activity, it would be very easy to argue that Martin's future world is now upon us. Contemporary research published in *Psychosomatic Medicine* in 2009 shows that an aggregate of leisure time well spent in activities such as socializing, spending quiet time alone, communing with nature, participating in sports or club activities, and visiting others is associated with positive mood and lower levels of the stress hormone cortisol. Two other recent studies have clearly demonstrated that the screen may be the antithesis of a leisure-time health promoter. Specifically, researchers found that regardless of physical activity and physical functioning, screen use during leisure time is associated with diminished mental well-being and higher levels of psychological distress in both children and adults.

---

### Vitamin G Extra Strength—the Mindfulness Factor

Cyberspace is the great distraction ... it follows the hiker into the wilderness and diverts attention from the then-and-there. Like life-giving water, cyberspace helpfully insinuates itself into the crevices of reality only to erode what it has promised to nurture.

—*Professor Albert Borgmann*

Mindfulness is the practice of paying attention to what you are experiencing in the current moment, remaining in the here and now without drifting off to the worry of the future or the experiences of the past. Mindfulness involves suspending judgment and letting go of opinions that would otherwise fire up the stress response. Nonjudgmental observation fosters acceptance, self-reflection, and greater ability to handle difficulties without avoidance. Mindfulness also enhances connectivity to nature, a critical ingredient in creating depth to otherwise superficial concerns for the environment.

In his 1942 textbook, dermatologist and University of Pennsylvania professor John H. Stokes provided advice to medical students and their patients. He recommended: "And one must focus the attention on things that take him [the patient] outside himself. Hence walking out of doors . . . watching the wind, the clouds, the grass and trees, or if in the city, the life about one is the proper method." This is vitamin G *extra strength* defined—the focused awareness of the detail in the leaves, the bark on the trees, the activities of insects, the movement of water.

The concept of mindfulness is not new, and its values have been discussed for centuries in various traditions, yet only recently has the scientific community evaluated the potential of mindfulness in health promotion. For example, Canadian research published in 2011 shows that among over 450 university students, mindfulness is highly linked to the associations between connectivity to nature and psychological well-being. The strength of research on the benefits of mindfulness on overall mental health has grown by leaps and bounds; however, the forte of mindfulness is its ability to remove *negative* thoughts from our cognitive equation. Vitamin G, simply being in and around greenspace, can promote *positive* thoughts. The end result of the combination— minimizing negativity and enhancing positivity through mindful greenspace experiences—is greater than the sum of the individual parts. We might consider mindful exercise in greenspace as vitamin G *triple strength*!

The solutions to the leisure problem can be found in at least small doses of vitamin G. To expand the potential of vitamin G's brain benefits in the context of a sustainable planet, to encourage people to really care about green, at least some semblance of identification with nature must be cultivated during leisure time. We need not become the next John Muir, Henry David Thoreau, or Gilean Douglas; however, if we can just step back from the screen for a bit and engage with nature, connect with the earth, there will be multiple benefits to all of us and the planet.

In a study published in 2009 in the *Journal of Health Psychology,* among almost 550 urban men and women, higher scores on the connectivity to nature scale were associated with greater overall psychological well-being, vitality, and—very importantly—meaningfulness. People scoring high on meaningfulness scales perceive themselves as living life with purpose, fulfillment, and satisfaction, and do not feel socially isolated. Meaningfulness is a marker of social connectivity, not social media connectivity. The more connected a person feels to nature, the greater the sense of meaningful involvement in something larger than oneself.

Canadian psychologist Elizabeth K. Nisbet, an expert in the relationship between one's relationship to nature and mental health, has reported that the strong connections between nature connectivity and personal well-being are found broadly in the population—from private-sector executives and high-ranking government employees to university students, the positive relationship is evident. Moreover, in a study published in 2011 in *Psychological Science,* Nisbet's Carleton University team showed that contact with nature can foster a positive mood state, which in turn facilitates a sense of nature relatedness. The researchers enrolled volunteers who were under the impression that they were involved in a study assessing personality and impressions of the campus area. In reality, the researchers were evaluating the psychological effects of walking different routes—one through buildings and tunnels and the other outdoors through mixed greenspace—to specific locations in and around the campus. Walking for just 15 minutes through greenspace, as expected, was associated with a more positive post-walk mental outlook. The more important discovery, something that ecotherapy experts have been concerned about for years, was that individuals were unable to forecast up front that taking differing indoor and outdoor routes could influence mood. A lack of anticipation of the benefits derived from urban nature helps to explain the behavioral avoidance of greenspace. Although the erosion of our connection to nature may be obscuring its perceived benefits, there is reason for optimism: critically, the researchers also showed that walking in nature lifted mood, and mood elevation via nature exposure appears to increase relatedness to nature. This is the happy-person, happy-planet cycle that can be maintained by provoking a little bit of nature identity. An individual can have many identities, and these are subject to change over time, yet the personal values that are placed on identity can have profound implications for health. For example, adults who begin to identify themselves as healthy will seek out more information on the nutritional quality of foods, consume more fruits and vegetables, and promote healthier eating habits in their children. People need to be made more aware of the psychological benefits of nature; education and vitamin G prescriptions can help with this process. Given the positive relationship between nature identity and conservation/pro-environmental attitudes, the experience of even nearby nature can, as Nisbet and her colleague Dr. John Zelenski suggest, open up a happy path to sustainability.

### Are You Nature Connected?

Researchers use a variety of psychological tests to evaluate the degree to which an individual might be connected to nature. For example, there is the Connectedness to Nature Scale, the Nature Relatedness Scale, and the Connectivity to Nature Scale. These scales are typically weighted around strength of agreement with statements such as:

- I feel a sense of oneness with nature.
- I enjoy the outdoors.
- I feel a personal bond with elements of the natural world, including plants and animals.
- My relationship to nature is an important part of my identity.
- My connection to animals, plants, and the earth influences my lifestyle.

- My well-being is connected to the well-being of the natural world.
- My actions can influence the health of the natural world.
- The self and nature are part of a continuous circle.
- Plants and wildlife require protection.
- I often go outdoors into nature.
- I enjoy leisure time in remote areas.

Researchers have shown that the strength of agreement with such questions can predict environmental concerns and actions.

---

### The Benefits of Volunteering for and within Nature

Mental health experts often recommend volunteering as a way to reduce stress and break the lure of sedentary life in front of a screen. Although it is unclear if all types of volunteerism are equally beneficial, we do know that environmental volunteering is associated with positive physical and mental health. Practical engagement in conservation volunteerism in natural settings provides opportunity for a dose of vitamin G, fosters a stronger nature identity, and expands social networks. A study published in 2011 in the *Journal of Environmental Psychology* showed that being outdoors in nature boosts vitality above and beyond the well-known benefits of physical activity and social interactions.

---

## Cities of the Future—*Vis Medicatrix Naturae* for All

> *I am a lover of knowledge, and in the city I can*
> *learn from men; but the fields and the trees can teach*
> *me nothing.*
> —Socrates, in *Phaedrus,* 360 BC

Cities can be wondrous hubs of inspiration, education, arts, commerce, culture, architecture, technology, and cohesiveness. Humans are incredibly social creatures, so it is not at all unnatural that urban centers should grow and thrive. Within the next several decades, our transition from rural to city life will be near complete, with some 90 percent of North Americans and 70 percent of global residents projected to call a city their home. There are, however, some alarming concerns with this inevitable trend. Compared with rural growth, urban population growth has been shown to drive deforestation and increase consumption of nutrient-depleted processed meats and other foods. It is incredibly inefficient to transport goods long distances for our cities, and the processing of foods for urban convenience is part of the so-called urban efficiency. Of course, there are also the concerns of crowding and lack of a place for green contemplation and mental rejuvenation. The research discussed in this book should inspire government officials, urban planners, and health-care professionals to be on top of their greenspace game. In particular, the recent findings on the mental health implications of urban biodiversity and brief exposure to city greenspace and its ability to influence nature connectivity should be taken into serious consideration. We cannot assume that this will happen. In September 2011, *Scientific American* devoted its entire issue to the bright future of better cities, and it did so with nary a mention of the importance of urban greenspace and forests to mental health and social justice within expanding cities, indicating that we have work to do. Collectively, we must ensure that our elected officials, our planners, and our mental-health-care providers are aligned in understanding the public health implications of a broad deficiency in vitamin G. They must understand that, as wonderful and awesome as cities might be, and with due respect to Socrates, the fields and trees can teach us plenty.

Access to parks and greenspace narrows the socioeconomic health inequality gap. Socially deprived urban schools are not surrounded by urban woodland; rather, they are belted by industrial zones, convenience stores, and clusters of fast-food outlets, so-called gray space—up to five and a half times more than in wealthier areas. For the schoolchildren who need it the most, dietary greens are off their plates and landscape greens are out of view. Cities need parks and greenspace not only as a means of encouraging physical activity; all of its citizenry, regardless of socioeconomic position, should be entitled to utilize the *vis medicatrix naturae,* to allow it to "minister to the mind," as Professor J. Arthur Thomson put it. Ultimately, the personal awareness of *vis medicatrix naturae* in positive psychology will win the hearts and minds of the populace in terms of conservation and sustainability—versus negative messaging wherein folks are more likely to feel disempowered and throw in the environmental towel.

By 2020, mental health disorders, depression in particular, are projected to be overwhelming health-care concerns, and cities are far from a panacea for depression. Indeed, rates of depression, anxiety, and schizophrenia are consistently reported to be much higher among urban residents than among their rural brethren. This takes us to the crux of the matter, the very reason we penned this book: there is no health without mental health. Our entire discussion, everything we have included in this book on the connection (and contemporary disconnection) between nature and brain health boils down to that phrase "No health without mental health." Although it is an official tagline of the World Health Organization and the United Kingdom's Royal College of Psychiatrists, it is not a mere slogan. Positive mental health is well upstream of most discussions of contemporary health-care problems. Mental health disorders affect the rates of countless other medical conditions, including communicable and noncommunicable diseases. When depression and anxiety creep into the mix of existing medical conditions, they serve to exacerbate the situation, and they also diminish help-seeking and adherence to healthy lifestyle habits. Anxiety and depression accelerate the aging of the human body; even when suicide is excluded, depression has been shown to increase the risk of premature mortality.

Technology—at least in its newly co-opted definition of screens, gadgets, and apps to make amusement more appealing—has not served to slow the tide of mental health disorders. Greater urban access to $5 latte shops has not stemmed the tide of the mental health crisis, nor will it. We require upstream solutions in the form of preventive variables, and vitamin G is proving itself to be a mental nutrient of prevention. Recall there is a trucker climbing into the well-appointed cab of a semi-trailer right now, as many more will in the future, to deliver a pharmaceutical elixir to an increasingly anxious, nature-detached, and depressed populace. It might seem irrelevant if he or she is hauling heavier loads of Prozac to future cities in a more fuel-efficient rig! Futurists are entitled to dream about better and brighter cities teeming with technological advancements, more screens and bar-code scanners in more places, fast food served up at a faster pace, theme park–like places where residents are propelled merely by the ever-increasing efficiency of so-called cyber-connectivity. However, by ignoring earth connectivity, modern nature disconnection, mental health, and its association with actual living greenspace, the techno-cratic optimism might be dashed on its plastic-resin rocks.

## Step Out of the Blogosphere and into the Atmosphere

While we can't say for sure what John Muir's opinion would be on infotoxicity, it seems evident he favored action over words and more words: "No amount of word-making will ever make a single soul to know these mountains." With the right amount of awareness and cautionary planning, the glass remains more than half full. As we con-clude this book, full circle in many ways, we are filled with optimism. Although the magnetic lure of the screen and infotoxins continue to exist as powerful undertows, scientific research is beginning to shed light on the dual problem of screen overload and nature withdrawal. Some of the most exciting studies in the area of excessive screen time and nature as medicine, and the implications of these forces, have been published only very recently. With awareness, policy makers, planners, and health-care providers can place appropriate signage: be careful of the undertow while swimming in technology. We can also provide much-needed life preservers in the form of vitamin G. We are hopeful that we are in the midst of a shift, the kindling of scientific awareness of vitamin G as propelled by a variety of exciting studies conducted by multiple branches of medicine. The isolated work of a few scientists involved in the nature-human relationship is now spreading to become the collective interest of frontline health-care providers. In order to sway our health-care providers, planners, and politicians, we need more than the words of Thoreau. We live in the age of science; therefore, we must provide scientific evidence that nature is a medicinal force, and indeed that is now happening. We suspect that researchers have now turned a corner in the scientific evaluation of vitamin G, with volumes of research to follow on both its effective dosage forms and the implications of deficiency.

Our optimism extends to the expanding future of our cities. The increasing use of rooftop trees and other vegetation is pleasing to look at, encourages biodiversity, and provides environmental advantages. Community gardens are an essential way to maintain earth-connectivity and are poised to experience a continued growing trend. Yet, living roofs and community gardens are not walkable parks. To have better and greener cities, we need more vegetation-dense parks teeming with biodiversity. Cities will boost creativity and positively influence the well-being of its citizenry by planting more trees in more places and by developing urban forests and urban national parks. It is hardly by chance that the happiest cities on earth are those that have an expansive waistline—a large greenbelt, that is. It has been said that national parks were "America's best idea," and we can now envision a day when the expansion of urban forests, greenbelts, and core greenspace in our cities will be North America's "even better idea."

In 1968, Dr. Edward Stainbrook, chair of the Department of Psychiatry, University of Southern California School of Medicine, said:

*Just to be in frequent perceptual contact with the reassuring, enduring earth is a psychological security factor of considerable importance . . . it is only as man can confidently, securely and exultantly reprocess his own nature and the greater nature of what we know as the world that he remains resourcefully in the directing vanguard of his own destiny. That is where the slowly evolving changes of nature have placed him. We can only go with nature and with our feet pressed against the earth. Otherwise we may follow the Pied Piper of our materialism and technology to the desperate edge of our increasingly plastic and synthetic existence.*

One wonders if the technocratic planners of today were planning New York City or Vancouver from scratch, would they devote such valuable land to Central Park and Stanley Park? We hope they would. Second chances are rare, and experience shows that it takes tremendous amounts of work by nature-conscious citizenry and environmental groups to undo urban planning conducted without greenspace in mind. Stainbrook was optimistic, as indeed we are, that humans can thrive as cities expand, as long as some earth-connectivity conditions are met through urban greenspace opportunities, which are so incredibly important at this time in human history. We close our book with his words, and a question of our own:

Did you get your vitamin G today?

# Appendix
# Resources

## References

A detailed, chapter-by-chapter list of the works cited in this book is available at the following website:
www.yourbrainonnature.com

## Authors

Eva M. Selhub, MD
www.drselhub.com

Alan C. Logan, ND
www.drlogan.com
www.vitaminG.com

## Natural and Holistic Medicine Organizations

International Society of Nature and Forest Medicine
www.infom.org

Benson-Henry Institute for Mind Body Medicine
151 Merrimac Street, 4th Floor
Boston, MA 02114
Phone: 617-643-6090
Fax: 617-643-6077
www.massgeneral.org/bhi

American Association of Naturopathic Physicians
4435 Wisconsin Avenue NW, Suite 403
Washington, DC 20016
Tel: 202-237-8150
Toll-free: 866-538-2267
Fax: 202-237-8152
www.naturopathic.org

Canadian Association of Naturopathic Doctors (CAND)
20 Holly Street, Suite 200
Toronto, ON M4S 3B1
Tel: 416-496-8633
Toll-free: 800-551-4381

Fax: 416-496-8634
www.cand.ca

American Holistic Medical Association
27629 Chagrin Boulevard, Suite 213
Woodmere, OH 44122
Phone: 216-292-6644
Fax: 216-292-6688
www.holisticmedicine.org

## Horticultural Therapy
American Horticultural Therapy Association
www.ahta.org

Canadian Horticultural Therapy Association
www.chta.ca

## Nutrition
Environmental Working Group
Provides up-to-date information on mercury in fish, and pesticides on produce.
1436 U Street NW, Suite 100
Washington, DC 20009
Phone: 202-667-6982
www.ewg.org

International Fish Oil Standards
Nutrasource Diagnostics Inc.
Provides public disclosure of independent testing on commercial fish oil supplements.
120 Research Lane, Suite 203
University of Guelph Research Park
Guelph, ON N1G 0B4
Phone: 519-341-3367
Toll-free: 877-557-7722
www.nutrasource.ca

Genuine Health Inc.
317 Adelaide Street W, Suite 501
Toronto, ON M5V 1P9
Phone: 416-977-8765
Toll-free: 877-500-7888
www.genuinehealth.com

Oldways Preservation and Exchange Trust
266 Beacon Street
Boston, MA 02116
Phone: 617-421-5500
www.oldwayspt.org

## Research, Education, and Publications

Ancestral Health Annual Symposium
Provides an evolutionary perspective in the quest to develop solutions to our modern
health-care dilemmas.
www.ancestryfoundation.org

St. Philip's Academy
St. Philip's Academy (kindergarten to eighth grade) in Newark, New Jersey, provides
an excellent example of the ways in which urban education meets conservation,
contact with nature, nutritional awareness, and environmental perspectives.
www.stphilipsacademy.org/

*Ecopsychology*
Dr. Thomas J. Doherty, editor-in-chief
Lewis & Clark Graduate School of Education and Counseling
www.liebertpub.com

# About the Authors

**Eva M. Selhub, MD,** is a Clinical Associate of the Benson-Henry Institute for Mind Body Medicine at the Massachusetts General Hospital and an Instructor in Medicine at Harvard Medical School. Specializing in Comprehensive Medicine, she has a private practice in Waltham, Massachusetts. Dr. Selhub has lectured throughout the United States and Europe and has trained health-care professionals from all over the world. Dr. Selhub also works as an executive coach, helping professionals from all over the globe to optimize leadership skills and achieve even greater success. She is the author of *The Love Response* (Ballantine 2009) and she has been published in medical journals and featured in national publications including *The New York Times, USA Today, Self, Shape, Fitness,* and *Journal of Women's Health,* and has appeared on radio and television in connection with her work. She has several audio CDs offering guided meditations. For more information, you can visit her website at www.theloveresponse .com or www.drselhub.com.

**Alan C. Logan, ND,** is a naturopathic doctor, scientist, and independent researcher focusing on nutritional medicine and ecotherapy. He graduated magna cum laude from the State University of New York at Purchase, and as valedictorian from the Canadian College of Naturopathic Medicine in Toronto. He is currently invited faculty in the mind-body medicine courses in Harvard's School of Continuing Medical Education; his lectures include The Placebo and Dietary Supplements, Exploration of Food and Mood in Positive Psychology, and Vitamin G: The Medicinal Aspects of Green Space. He is author of *The Brain Diet* (2007) and co-author of several books within dermatology.

Dr. Logan has written extensively on the intriguing connection between the gut and mental health conditions (the so-called gut-brain axis) and even more recently on the gut-brain-skin axis. His commentaries have appeared in a wide variety of mainstream medical journals (from the *Archives of Dermatology* to the *Journal of Neurotrauma*) and in many popular magazines, including *Cosmopolitan, Elle, W, Health,* and *Life & Style*. For more information, you can visit his website at www.drlogan.com and www.vitaminG.com.

# Index